Dark Clouds Hide The Sun

John England

DARK CLOUDS HIDE THE SUN

Published by Memorial Publications, 2014
Copyright © 2014 John England
ISBN: 978-1501079047

John England asserts the moral right to
be identified as the author of this work

Cover and interior images: JaxEtta.com Photography

All rights reserved. No part of this publication may be reproduced, stored in a retrieval system, or transmitted in any form or by any means - electronic, mechanical, photocopying, recording or otherwise - without the prior written permission of the publisher.

JOHN ENGLAND

Preface

'Dark Clouds Hide the Sun'
I wasn't quite sure what to call it.

A not too prepossessing title really, but I wanted to convey that feeling one gets when everything is perfect on a bright sunny day and then, from nowhere, springs a dark thundercloud. The feeling too that is engendered in discovering footprints in wet concrete, or that when a pet dog rubs itself on a freshly painted door.

You see this is a true love story, of deep devotion and a union of mind and spirit in the true sense of those words. That lovely word contentment sums it up, or 'Soul Mates'. Indeed a phrase so often heard in a former TV ad said it all, 'We just want to be together'.

On the other hand it could signify the trauma of what is termed an eternal triangle where, as Princess Diana so neatly put it 'There were three of us in this marriage'. This though was no other real live person, but an entity, as in the biblical sense of the man who was possessed by the devil.

Likewise you could say that warfare figures. For there is conflict and struggle, for the unfolding situation demands strength, courage, fortitude and the determination not to be beaten.

It is also a first, for no one to my knowledge has described, in such detail, the progress of Alzheimer's with Lewy bodies. In fact it is an extension of the information that was provided to the Psychiatrist who was primarily concerned, for a case study he was preparing.

It is too, an expose of current thinking and attitudes. Of the certain shortcomings of the Medical Profession, Social Services and of the so called Care in the Community. Governmental attitudes too, have to change and for why?

Well let's put it this way: Let's say a strangler, or a rapist is on the loose. There have been three or four, perhaps five victims so far. Communities are in shock, the Media works overtime and the Police are over-stretched, with possibly the need of the military to give them assistance. Sadly it's an all too familiar story.

Dementia though gets little mention. Not only is it not understood, but more importantly much mis-understood, when its consequences are nothing less than an ongoing Nine Eleven! Yes I don't have to exaggerate. We are not talking of the three, four, or five cases I have mentioned, that quickly focus the attention of the Nation, but the 600,000 currently and shortly expected 800,000 souls to be afflicted with Dementia. Thus there is much sadness in this story too.

This task will be far beyond the scope of the charity organisations who only deal with the residue of this curse. It is time that we, as a Nation, and whatever Government we have, acts decisively once and for all. Too many people are dying a long and distorted death, day by day and week by week.

It really is a war and the casualties are mounting, so it's REALLY TIME THAT WE, AS A NATION, DID SOMETHING VERY POSITIVE ABOUT IT!

JOHN ENGLAND

Something to Remember

In no way is this madness -
- this is more a loss of life!

You are presumably sitting quite comfortably at this moment, so now is perhaps a good time to consider what capabilities you have at this moment in time and which you obviously take for granted? Quite a few, are there not? So let's now consider just how many are likely to be lost, during the progress of Dementia. A life sentence in prison takes away plenty of privileges, but nothing like these benchmarks of freedom, which are lost for someone like Mary, who had Alzheimer's with Lewy bodies.

So let's now consider them, I think you will be quite surprised: loss of privacy, dignity and independence. Constant companionship with husband, or wife. Loss of access to 99% of your possessions, also your home and its comforts. Loss of normal eyesight, that remaining being much distorted. Loss of all notion of time and place. The Freedom to go where you please, to have holidays and regular outings. Loss of memory of almost all former happenings. Loss of mobility other than for a few feet, with no opportunity to plan your life. Loss of being able to go out shopping in town, or its surroundings, to have regular contact with friends, to entertain, or be entertained. Loss of financial decisions and access to money. Loss of your garden, its sights and smells, the pleasure of reading, or pastimes such as knitting. Loss of the pleasure of cooking, or tending your plants. Add to that the long hours of loneliness and the feeling of being 'put away', or Imprisoned, which really you are!

Not very nice is it? So count your blessings and, for a moment, remember both those that have this affliction and particularly the husband or wife whose life too has been shattered. I think first and foremost, they in particular need a better deal, but if Dementia is not to overwhelm both families and the very fabric of society; Governments of any hue must soon take drastic action. This scourge will never be conquered by having to rely on charitable donations for research into a cure. Government funding for that must now be a priority, so that the work of charities can be focused on easing the load of Carers.

Also these extremely important points -
- which must not be forgotten!

Within those afflicted there is no loss of love that can be bestowed, of tenderness, or kindness that is shown. No loss of the understanding of truth, honesty and decency. The ability to acknowledge kindness is retained, as is that of humour, friendship and courtesy. Nature, art, design and music too are greatly appreciated and there is awareness that apology is necessary, for behaviour that is demonstrated to be untoward. In other words, the person is totally normal in a great variety of important ways, retaining the ability to spot mistakes, even solve puzzles and when you are stuck for a word; provide either it, or a suitable alternative!

And all that and very much more my friend, is anything but mad.

JOHN ENGLAND

An Introduction

My name is unimportant, but for convenience I'll say it is John. The experience though perhaps is and it may serve as a warning of what you may face if you become a Carer, but most of all it will provide an accurate situation report, on not only what can be encountered, but open a window on what is largely unknown regarding the seemingly non-understanding and somewhat unco-ordinated 'Services' which are supposedly there to assist you. As you read on you will no doubt think I have a jaundiced view, but I have no axe to grind and do tell the truth, so I have decided to put this in writing as a warning and also in hope that it will see the light of day, someone might take note and seek to ensure that some other soul doesn't fare the same. However, if that is the outcome and a report be resultant, will anyone really take notice? I doubt it, for in this material world of today, in which we find ourselves, the key word seems to be 'Self', or perhaps 'Self Preservation' where officialdom is concerned. Some too may say that what is contained herein should not be published, for it would possibly cause increased anxiety to those so diagnosed. I do not agree, for forewarned is forearmed, is it not?

It is a personal account and as such just one of many thousands, all very different, but seldom does one read other than a few specific cases reported from time to time in newspapers to highlight some particular debacle. As I say, all individual cases are no doubt different, for the manner of disability covered by Carers is manifold and where Alzheimer's is concerned, this present day scourge is one understands, of somewhat limitless variation. As such you enter at the deep end, for few understand its full ramifications and as yet even fewer have the knowledge, or training to be of real use. This, I believe, unfortunately relates in particular to some General Practitioners. How long this will take to rectify is unknown, for much depends on not only funding, but a will by Government to truly realise the developing situation and what will be needed to manage it. Too much of this I suspect, is due to recent years when mental health underwent great change of emphasis, from the provision of monolithic Mental Hospitals, to so called Care in the Community.

This no doubt has advantages in regard to some, for being locked away and institutionalised no doubt blighted many lives that might have had opportunity to be brightened and an individual was not given opportunity to enjoy the wider world than that of four walls. I claim to be no expert, with only the simplest understanding of mental health, but I am a retired engineer and one who views my body and its various functions, in similar vein to mechanical systems and their reliability, or malfunctioning. In other words one who learns that to be able to form a valid strategy one must observe, note and collate one's findings to advantage. For example, throughout my childhood, but two doors away from my home, the mother of one of my school friends took in washing and provided board and lodging to commercial travellers, in an endeavour to make ends meet throughout the 1930s; while her husband, a former soldier of the Great War, remained long years in a large mental home nearby, one of three at that time within some twenty miles of each other.

It would take the onset of a further war before he was allowed out for odd days, a freedom that was gradually increased, until somewhat surprisingly he became a member of the Home Guard and as such was in charge, as a Sergeant if I remember correctly; of a local equipment store where weapons and ammunition were regularly in his sole charge. Thus if that example is anything to go by, perhaps one can judge that the aforementioned release from four walls, where possible, was a constructive enterprise, however today I fear saving money is what drives what I would term Social Engineering and even though many care homes are little more than an extension of that earlier four wall situation, staying at home is the far better option. Capital is made by officialdom on stating the 'bleeding obvious', that by and large couples do not want to be separated; but this fiction of conscience, so widely promoted, obscures their finding that it is far cheaper for National and local government to pay out allowances and let someone else carry the can.

All too convenient, but there are casualties with this system and in my experience, they are mostly unrecognised and largely ignored. No doubt by now you are saying this is a rare case, for things are wonderful aren't they? Well you will have to judge for yourself if you choose to read on, but we're not all Terry Pratchett's; whose much publicised TV programmes didn't bear the slightest relationship to my experiences and neither, I doubt, to many others. If anything, he being well-known, with his Alzheimer's in its early stages and having the means at his disposal, it was a rather too public experimentation, by one who could easily afford his own full time Carer, almost like a personal assistant. I suspect that 'Care' overall doesn't get enough 'warts and all' exposure, for there can be few who have the time to record detail. I've started this now as a result of encountering a dose of uncaring officialdom and heaven knows if I will ever finish it, but someone needs to adopt this procedure, for there's presently a lot of papering over the cracks and loads of expensive publications around that to the casual observer seem to meet every requirement. Politicians of all parties constantly make promises and love whatever photo opportunity they can engender, only to move on to further sound bites and more of the same. Look at any local authority vacancy list, the salaries are fairy tale if the world you were brought up in was Pounds, Shillings and Pence.

When these 'social engineers' are encountered, they are invariably young, well-dressed, polite, freshly schooled, but with little experience of life and many of the older ones no better, listening, making notes and making promises, yes, lots of promises that mostly prove to be nothing more than fresh air and as I hope to show, it all leaves you feeling pretty helpless!

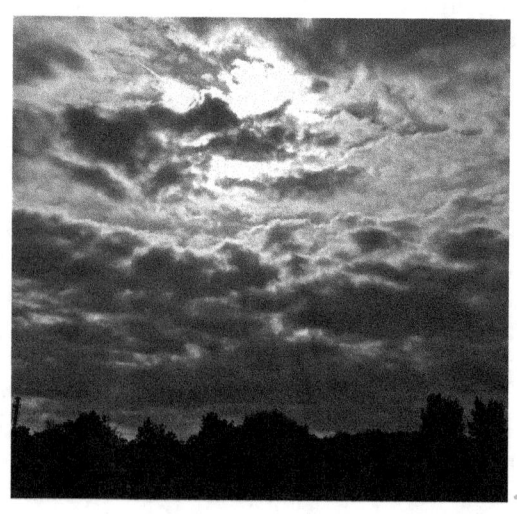

JOHN ENGLAND

The Origins

So when did this particular experience originate and what has happened along the way since that time? In actual fact the first instance was quite a few years back and so unusual, that it was months before I realised why it could have happened, putting it down to a moment of unsureness on the part of my wife (who I will call Mary), whilst in the company of complete strangers.

The occasion back in the year 2000, was a visit to a couple at a nearby town, where the man wanted to purchase one of my self-published books and while he and I chatted on that subject, his wife engaged Mary in a pleasant and relaxed general conversation. Indeed it was a very pleasant occasion; one thing led to another and in passing the lady happened to ask Mary her Christian name. Something that would have received instant and almost automatic response; but fact was she couldn't say it, she couldn't remember it and it was so unbelievable, that the silence ensuing was truly embarrassing. However, there would be no recurrence for several months and that moment, in ignorance, was lost without realisation of what the future was to bring.

Instead it was many and unassociated other medical reasons that were to take precedence, such as fainting and a long term heart difficulty associated with palpitations. The late summer of a later year saw too the commencement of sight problems, initially of pain in the eye, leading to laser surgery and eventual replacement of the lens in both eyes, not so much for cataracts, but as a method of easing the build-up of pressure in the eyes, which had been the cause of pain. A further complication then arose in respect of double and treble vision, plus other obscuration which persists today and is of greater magnitude, despite the best efforts of our local hospital.

By now the need for myself to undertake the bulk of household tasks was also necessitated through increasing loss of Mary's mobility and my being of increasing years, I felt it was time to ask for assistance. It took a bit of doing and perhaps for too long I had resisted what might be termed, 'throwing in the towel' and asking for help from the local authority's Social Services. It was certainly not done easily, for my being an independent soul and ever managing on basic pension, I would have chosen to continue likewise.

As pressure mounted I eventually decided to make a call and after all of the questions from a lady of obvious foreign accent were answered; I waited patiently for some response. Days became weeks and I began to wonder if I would ever hear further. Could this be normal procedure, I wondered? Meanwhile various visits to surgery continued for a range of upcoming and ongoing reasons and in the course of these, no fewer than two hasteners were submitted on my behalf by its nursing staff. This being so, there was still no response, even though I was to learn much later that my initial call had been logged as dangerous and those that followed from the surgery were categorised as urgent! By chance at that time a leaflet of a political party arrived through the post, within which somewhat conveniently included space to identify any subject that in one's opinion required attention. I accepted the offer and duly notified the sender of further detail, he being a local councillor, who it turned out also had a seat on the local County Council.

Now with all the relevant detail, I imagine he duly brought the matter up, for in due course I did receive an apology, although it plainly consisted of a lengthy diatribe of no sincerity whatever, as if an off-the-shelf selection to be issued when relevant. With great suspicion that it would have been taken to heart and procedures perhaps changed, I reported back to him, sensing that he appeared to share my feelings. When several of its sentences were read out over the phone, it certainly prompted him to wish to borrow it for greater scrutiny. I agreed to the request, saying nevertheless I did want to retain it for the record, but when I later took it to his home, I was to find that all contact ended. He kept the letter and has never contacted me further from that day to this. So much for politicians in general and their promises, whatever the party!

Meanwhile, where Mary was concerned, did I but realise it, there were isolated instances to indicate the loss of knowing one's own name was not just a chance aberration, but an isolated indicator of the initial step; in a process that would in time have all the ingredients to destroy a happy marriage and most certainly put an end to the life which we had enjoyed until that time. In themselves they were innocent little things that arose, even giving rise to banter about the onset of old age and statements like needing to wake oneself up. Several were forgetting to buy a newspaper on various day's visits to town and one late return was to reveal Mary getting on the wrong bus for the return to home and thereby ending up on the other side of town.

Anyway, none were that dramatic that they couldn't be rectified and increasing age was blamed, for I too, being around five years younger, was beginning to find I had to keep a note of things and tick them off once they had been completed. There were too several falls, initially thought to be connected with failing vision and increasing frailty, but they necessitated yet more surgery visits and great reliance on myself to minimise the risk of their reoccurrence. This I was more than happy to do, for as one who had lived alone for several years following an earlier marriage, I had no difficulty where meals were concerned and any job related to garden and home maintenance came easily to one well used to being self-reliant.

An Early Warning

Indeed this was second nature for subsequent to a childhood with little, or no schooling through illness, it took effort to work my way up to the holding of responsible positions with nationally known companies, where integrity and precision was prime requirement. During these early days the Alzheimer's aspect, was by far the lesser reason to undertake the bulk of household management; I could on rare occasion continue to have a day away with my son over to the continent, two or three times a year, taking the advantage of some 'silly' air fares then available with a well-known carrier and approaching one year's end, this increased to a special overnight in Germany.

I departed confident that all would be well, for despite the aforementioned problems, Mary remained capable and the only downside was that I would not be with her on her birthday. The enjoyable break complete, it was of no great concern that a call home had not been picked up, for she might well have been taking a nap, but upon our landing, I was eager to advise her that I would be home before long. Thus my son rang, but again there was no reply. Doubt filled me. Something must be wrong, he had better ring his mother to see if she knew what might be the reason, for she had arranged to keep in contact with Mary whilst we were away. It was, as by that time I expected, bad news! Mary had been taken into hospital early the previous morning, but this was no normal admission. She had been found fallen in the road and in a distressed state, in the early hours of the morning by a nurse living opposite.

Relaying the first details to me, my son then made what turned out to be a very profound statement, by saying, "I think that's the last time you'll be going anywhere for a long time!" When I reached home ahead of going to the hospital, it was very obvious that all was not well. The normally tidy room was in some disarray, with clothing scattered around and papers likewise, as if something had been searched for and venturing upstairs, I found the situation repeated. On arrival at the hospital and directed to a ward, I was to find someone I almost didn't recognise, ashen faced, confused, hair bedraggled and untidily dressed!

Mary didn't look any different to a disaster victim and couldn't tell me anything really coherent as to what had befallen her, neither too could the hospital staff. My overwhelming need was to take her away from there and get her home as soon as possible, but that was easier said than done, for gathering up her belongings was a problem and nobody seemed to want to help. To this day I'm sure items of clothing had gone missing, never to be seen again, but get Mary home I did and try to get to the bottom of what had gone so desperately wrong in so short a time.

During the next day or so I was gradually able to piece together what had happened and it, like so many other things later, was a salutary learning of things encountered during life; that we were never told about at school, or at any other time for that matter. I was to eventually ascertain that the first overnight had been normal. Next day this continued in a phone conversation with my former wife during the evening prior to the hospitalisation and also Mary's friend in a neighbouring town. From there on it becomes difficult to understand exactly, but at some time during that night confusion and terror had arrived to overwhelm Mary, with horrible figures present that drove her to frantically get together some basic possessions, before driving her out from the house. It seems she was heading out seeking to catch a bus back to where she had previously lived in another town.

Her flight, however, from these demons ended only yards from the front door, for she tripped on a kerb (we think) and cut open her leg in the process, to lay calling out for help in the gutter. Awful as this was, it seems it was not yet a manifestation of the oncoming Alzheimer's condition, for this would not be for a further eight or so months yet; but this time it was something far more simple. Naturally there was further contact with Mary's doctor, who in a very matter of fact way said, "It was simply the result of a water infection". When I expressed my surprise, she said it was quite common for this to bring about confusion, but it had never done so before, or did for long after, thank goodness.

Once we were together and at home, Mary was fine again in no time, with the episode quickly gone, yet not forgotten. We carried on as usual, with the calendar used to mark off the various recurring hospital and surgery appointments quickly giving the appearance that most weeks were, shall we say, dominated by things that just had to be done, which left little time for anything else. It was in fact the first stages of an incarceration that would in due course intensify. Even though there was now severe limitation to where we could go and what we could do as far as any holiday, or visit to an event was concerned, I did finally manage to arrange a very pleasant break.

Despite lack of mobility, sensory deprivation and this ever present dizziness or faintness we finally made the effort and were able to enjoy a fortnight's holiday in the Gloucestershire area, which did we but realise it, would be our last. By now both hips and knees were adding to the difficulty substantially and agreement was obtained for the replacement of a right hip. This part of the story would perhaps be a suitable time to recount something regarding the provision of aids to mobility.

In general terms this had to be described as good, however there was one exception as will be seen later. As a consequence of an exploratory visit to our home, things like handrails, bath steps, perch seat and the provision of heightening for chairs and another special chair, were either fitted, or supplied readily. Other than this, zimmer frames and commodes for upstairs and down were provided, along with separate personal instructional visits in regard to the best way to provide physical support without incurring injury to oneself in the process.

Much of this was related to the intended admission to hospital for the hip replacement and there was also hospital attendance to thoughtful instruction of both the mechanics of the operation and procedures needed subsequently, during the important post-operative period. Here though was the exception to this, for hospital procedures utilised a post-op three step trial piece with handrail and this of course bore no comparison with tackling the stairs in your average semi, with a winder three quarters of the way up. With a hip op only, perhaps, but this was also a patient with persistent dizziness and visual disability, so could a stair lift perhaps be obtained?

Not readily came the answer, for if I remember this was June and I was notified, that consideration was apparently only now being undertaken for applications made in April of the previous year! Faced with this, it seemed there was little hope and nothing else for it than for Mary to be taken upstairs upon return from hospital and remain there. In taking up the request of the hospital to procure several other post-op aids that would be of use and also thinking in terms of a rotatable pad to assist in car travel, I paid a visit to a health care shop to purchase these and there enquired perchance, of what a privately purchased stair lift might cost, being well aware that the daily newspaper ads seen are careful not to mention this and that it could well be beyond my means.

This was certainly so, but the kindly proprietor, upon asking and being told the details, said he might well be able to help! He revealed that he was on the committee of a charity that I had not heard of and was prepared to make a submission on my behalf at the next week's meeting; if I quickly obtained a couple of quotes and completed the required paperwork.

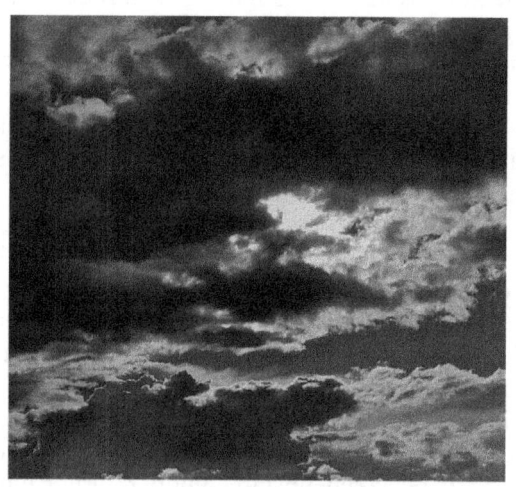

The Death of Expectations

This was then done with due haste and I was greatly pleased to find soon after, that my part payment offered had been matched twice over, with the result that two thirds of the cost would be provided to my assistance. It was indeed a Godsend, for the two local officials who had visited earlier had been most insistent, in saying that a bed must be moved downstairs, something that in a lounge diner in full view of the road, would have been most impractical. However, where the stair lift was concerned, it wasn't the end of the story by far, but more of that at a later stage of this story.

Where the intended operation was concerned, it all seemed straight forward enough and we were then blissfully ignorant that early Alzheimer's would be diagnosed in a matter of days following admission. Likewise we were completely unaware that this was likely to dramatically escalate with any change of lifestyle, such as holiday let alone hospitalisation, even be it temporary. True there had been an attendance at the Memory Clinic back in May where a gentleman doctor had been most considerate, but it had only involved some testing and the acquisition of general background information, for he obtained reasonable results from a memory test and things had yet to be a cause of any great concern.

This being so, and we having had no break of any kind for ages, I went ahead with plans for the holiday to be in the Gloucestershire area. It was thus completed around nine months after my ill-fated weekend trip to Germany and thankfully all went well, allowing for the mobility difficulties in particular. Despite that area then having just experienced the twin perils of flooding and water shortage, the sun thankfully shone upon us and it proved to be most enjoyable. It was planned to encompass all the things we had both traditionally enjoyed doing and as such, typified our time together until then, but sadly it was to be our last, for as I have intimated in a matter of just a few weeks later, the Alzheimer's would put an end to life as we had previously known it.

Notified that a bed would be free during the third week of September, the preliminaries were completed and we looked forward to an increase in Mary's mobility. However, it only took a matter of hours once she entered hospital, to find this was not to be, for I was to find she had been moved from the general ward into a side room, so as hopefully to be more visible to the nursing staff, due to her now becoming confused and prone to wandering. In time sadly there would be more to it than that and day by day the situation became far more complicated. The isolated falls that had occurred previously rapidly increased, especially in the aftermath of the operation, successful as it was; for confusion increased and no doubt for good reason, it wasn't possible for her to be watched all the time.

Mary's unhappiness now deepened, when rather than the expected few days on the ward, these had to be extended due to the picking up of one, or more, infections. After what seemed a lifetime, although checking back it was not much longer than a fortnight, she was allowed home. This in fact was to turn out to be a short visit rather than a homecoming, for within forty-eight hours the visit of a nurse to remove stitches, immediately brought about a disaster!

As it happened it was clips rather than stitches for removal, however it only took one look by myself to exclaim to this nurse, "I'm sorry, but I wouldn't take those out if I were you", for it was clear to see that several inches of the wound looked distinctly unsound and thus likely not to have knit together sufficiently. Despite my protestations she went ahead, for she supposedly knew better than I and removed all but around three in an eight to nine inch wound and totally undeterred by my comment, left us. As I busied myself in the kitchen with things that were needed regarding the preparing of a meal, only some ten minutes had elapsed before there was noisy commotion upstairs and a frantic cry for help.

Hurrying upstairs, I was confronted by the sight of Mary standing at the foot of the bed with blood spurting everywhere, clothing, bedclothes and floor, all bearing witness to the fact that things were seriously amiss. It was immediately clear too, that I could not cope with a situation like this and I quickly dialled 999. There was rapid response by a paramedic, who on arrival at the scene, took one look and immediately rang for an ambulance.

Asked by his controller presumably, to state what the situation was, he chose his words well, by saying; "She's stood here filling her slippers with blood!", for there was little better way to describe it! From then on, actions followed rapidly for her removal back to hospital and this event and what followed, only magnified the initiation of the Alzheimer's condition and its routines, if one can call them that. Unfortunately it was seemingly not appropriate for Mary to return to the original ward, where she had had good care overall and some provision had been possible of someone to sit with her. This time I was to find she had been placed in a trauma ward, where much too much activity and shortage of staff, precluded any close observation.

By the second day there were more falls, she was seeing terrifying demon faces on the walls of the room around her and I was asked to sit with her in the morning and to extend my visiting time of afternoon and evening substantially. This I did most willingly, but as one might understand, it extended a traumatic situation, for I had to grab what meal I could, while my presence did little, or nothing to ease her mental condition and the falls continued unabated. Every time I went she was to be found terrified and crying, while one of the afternoon visits was particularly harrowing for us both.

Upon entering the room, I was to find her barricaded up in the corner by the bed, plus whatever else could have been found at the time, in an attempt to make her comply with the need to stay in bed. The infection too was not easily conquered, for she kept pulling out the drips and other fittings attached to her body and I began to face the possibility of what our future life might be, if this episode should prove to be ongoing. The tension must have shown on my face, for one lady who was responsible for the return of patients to their home environment correctly, was more than helpful.

Aware that I knew little of what I was in for and was also completely unprepared, she not only found the time to photocopy every page of a book on Alzheimer's, but also wheeled Mary over to an appointment in the memory clinic we had previously attended. On arrival she agreed to stay with us throughout the meeting with a lady doctor, who again was most considerate. Both this lady and the doctor, through their kindness, helped me to confront this great unknown which until that time had meant so little. In truth it would take time to come to terms with the new situation and realisation in particular dawned that this was terminal, although not stated as such; for there was no cure and one never got better.

This instance, with others encountered both before and after with trained personnel who have practical skills, rather than theoretical knowledge; highlights the great difference that exists among those met along the way. This chasm between those who are trained and have understanding and those who believe they are important and have no compassion; to my mind detracts from one's task of caring. In that the latter have no real inkling of what is involved and dedication required, being hindrance, even source of aggravation rather than help, thus adding great frustration as one encounters an exacting regime of happenings and complications.

Early encounters if I can prove the point, included a man from an organisation, who listened, took notes and promised assistance in providing in the main simple answers as to where aid might be forthcoming, such as was there anywhere that Mary might have a bath; she now being unable to use the one at home. After some couple of hours he produced a questionnaire. Had I found his visit of assistance and had he conducted it to my satisfaction? Of course at that stage he had, so I was willing to give all the answers to his questionnaire that he was no doubt hoping for. But from the time he left there was no further contact, so that later and without a single answer; I felt I had been conned.

Indeed it was little different to another occasion when I had sought information much earlier from one of their town centre shops and again I was to leave empty handed. At another visit from another organisation's representative, my not being on the Internet seemed to be a problem, so I asked if there was any chance of learning where Mary might get a bath and might I be given copy of where toilets for the disabled were to be found in my home county. Again I felt I should have saved my breath, for few of the leaflets that arrived much later were of any real help and in regard to the toilets, there was only a short list of already known toilets in my own town!

Along the way too, a great deal was made of how one could take control, under a direct payments scheme of the local county council; whereby one had the chance to arrange care and support with a cash allowance. Its stated advantage was that being self-regulated, it could be tailored more exactly to one's needs. On the face of it, it sounded good, or perhaps a little too good, for nagging thought was, that wasn't this yet more of doing someone's work for them? However, I said I wanted more detail and this time not one, but two gents came and sat the seemingly regulation couple of hours, explaining little and left me really none the wiser.

I certainly understood the thought behind this initiative (as well as my sneaking suspicion), for if I were a young man, or woman who was maybe working and keeping contact at a distance from say a relative, I would have the time and necessary contacts to manage such an arrangement. Should this be so advertisements could be placed, interviews held, contracts could be offered and bank accounts opened. Also, I would know enough persons to be referees and arrange their audit of my transactions. Fine! ... but we do not have the necessary friends and relations, plus it took me all my time to fit in a haircut every second month, I was then approaching eighty and on duty, if you want to put it that way, what is now known as 24/7.

I very much wished I could do it, but I simply could not! With everything appertaining to two lives to remember those past three years, failing health and a failing memory of my own, I was increasingly unable to cope as well as I wished. When I said this all I got as reply was "You either do it yourself, or you lose it" and this despite the glossy pamphlets proclaiming - "It's your choice". "If not we will do it for you, or help you in every way." So was I not conned again? Returning to my story after this brief letting off of steam, I'll say one certainly has to do this every so often, else I'd have given up long ago, even though it doesn't do a lot to help at that moment.

However I did have a reputation in work days of having infinite patience, so even now I can bounce back from stressful times, ever hopeful. Eventually, after several frustrating postponements, I was allowed to bring Mary home from hospital and began an up and down stairs routine for everything that was required, for as yet the stair lift remained undelivered. As each visit was made in relation to the quotations from various companies, health and safety had reared its ugly head.

The straight lift, which I thought would be most suitable, was, I was told, no longer available. The stairs themselves were stated to be too narrow and this installation not for an old house, but one built in the 1950s. Also at first it was said it couldn't be fitted to the wall where one would expect, but only to the woodwork. This latter statement seemed somewhat ridiculous, for at the stair-head it would leave no room, blocking bedroom door entrances, whilst at base it would obstruct the hallway and block access to a meter cupboard.

A matter certainly to be frowned upon by not only meter readers, but likewise the power providers. Such was the problem it seemed (to them), that at one stage it was said one manufacturer wouldn't even countenance fitting it. The desire for money wasn't that underrated though by another and in due course the provision was accepted, except that two conditions must be agreed to and met. Firstly the stair lift must only be used under the control of myself using the remote and all the woodwork adjoining, must receive alteration to make it comply with clearance regulations. This was certainly not an overnight job, and at that stage I didn't fancy the additional costs that employing a builder/carpenter might incur; so there was no option, but to try and find the time to do this work myself!

Some Major DIY

No problem there, for I had a proven history of major do it yourself work over many years and had received praise for the standard of its completion, but that was when I had time to spare! Not daunted by the prospect, although another said I would never finish it, I commenced nigh on eight months, of a half hour here and three quarters there, as time allowed, until the work was completed. It too was complicated, by the requirement that at any time, the removal of any portion which was to undergo change, had to have immediate fitment of temporary safeguard.

Nevertheless the stair lift was finally installed, to commence a twelve month period of frequent malfunction, which would eventually require the assistance of Trading Standards, but more on that later also. With Mary home and this time thankfully for a more substantial period, the several weeks leading to Christmas saw her regain strength and within the home environment, revert to the person I had known previous to her two stays in hospital. A programme of therapy commenced with daily exercises and there was a visit by a continence nurse in the light of slight difficulty at night, due to initial restriction of movement. Where falls were concerned, although now restricted due to constant supervision, they did regrettably still feature.

JOHN ENGLAND

The Loss of Freedom

The most spectacular was early one morning in the bathroom, when both of us crashed down, demolishing a large plastic clothes basket in the process, myself also hitting my shoulder on a radiator! I think that brought the total to twenty-two, but it was the twenty-third while correctly using the zimmer on the Boxing Day evening, that Mary managed to fall in the hallway and among other things, also hit her head on a radiator. Since that time and for around thirteen months thankfully there were no others, for imagination, or not, it appeared to be the reason for another rapid acceleration in the Alzheimer's condition.

It may too have been aggravated by the so called Sundown, or Sunset Syndrome, where the dark nights appear to have some correlation to behaviour, but the onset was almost as pronounced as that upon her entry to hospital. From that fall until the following Easter, the nights were a source of torment to us both. Not only was there an increase in loss of short time memory, but almost a total loss of that for around the previous twenty years of her life.

Tragic as this was for Mary, it might not have been as bad had that period not encompassed several dramatic events. By dramatic I say things which are understood to be as markers, or stress points in one's life. In Mary's case it was not one, but several. First the death of her father, then an unhappy marriage and the loss of her only baby in its first hour. Later there would be the loss of a much loved step-father and finally her mother. A subsequent divorce from that difficult marriage, a later move from house to a flat, then our own marriage and the move to our present home.

I think it hard to imagine so many in so short a time and both then and now for that matter, she is lost, without answers to where she really is and believes either that certain of those events have only just happened, never did, or that her mother in particular is still alive. The situation is compounded that when one tries to tell her what little I know (for much was obviously long before we met); I am not believed and if I am, that knowledge is lost almost immediately, giving rise to the same questions being repeated over and over again! You will have to try to imagine the scenario, during the evenings of that winter and that wasn't all of it, for on many days it didn't commence at dusk, that is to say mid-afternoon, but at noon, or even earlier.

At this point, it is relevant to state that I have been led to believe by word and mouth, that when such situations arise it is recommended that one agrees to the sufferer's requests to do this and that, or promises it will be done in a minute, in the hope that it will then be forgotten. I can understand this might be appropriate where mundane things are the subject of the moment and the person is 'that far down the road' that they accept what is said, but where Mary is concerned this is certainly of no use.

At that time and even much later, she retained so much of her faculties, that visitors to our home, or who would then see Mary whilst out, would see only her frailty and related sight and mobility limitations. More importantly that high proportion of normality, apart from memory, didn't hinder conversation, or thoughtful discussion and she and I agree we continue the bond of mutual trust, whereby truth is pre-eminent. She said from the very start that she didn't want excuses, or lies and should they be detected it would end her trust in me, something most important when one considers her past and when she now relies on me to such a great extent.

Increasing Isolation

Not only that, but it would be totally against my nature, for trust and integrity were cornerstones of all my employments, to an unusual standard. Even so, when Mary would demand to be taken to her mother and property where she once lived, believing it was yesterday, or even a few hours earlier, such was just not possible and no excuse could, or ever will answer that particular demand. I will and have done many things I didn't think possible, but I cannot raise the dead, even if I wished! However, believe me there were, and remain, countless occasions where after several hours of confrontation I only just wished I could, for that particular and ever recurring facet of her present distress remained over the years a daily occurrence!

Many daylight hours as I have said were at that time still almost normal and with the day's routine tasks completed with the preparation of the main meal, its consumption and washing up done, my hope throughout was for the chance for a couple of evening hours of rest. The start of the six o'clock news commenced this hoped for period, with a favourite TV programme to maybe follow and if not, the watching perhaps of a DVD. If it turned out to be a bad night, I might be lucky for an hour, or so, before the Alzheimer's kicked in and when it did, it was and remains very easily recognised. In my head the alarm bells would ring, not knowing if it was to be a short, or long haul before an enforced early retirement might be one means of bringing it to conclusion.

The closing of the eyes and a loss of attention herald the start, or the head is seen to be looking elsewhere in the room and one knows that any moment now the first of those questions will begin. Some evenings it would start with a question about the people who had tea with us (none did), or with reference to another who had supposedly been sitting on the settee earlier. Others that followed were most likely to relate to unfinished business, such as clothing, keys, furniture, curlers, medicines that have come to mind, as being left behind and thus it was a situation needing action. Other variations then related to persons such as her mother, or an imagined old man in a wheelchair, who she must get back to, having left them earlier as if one was on a visit to me.

Although we never left the house after dark, there was also suddenly a need to put on coat and shoes. If I said what are you looking down there for, it was because a book, or whatever had appeared on the floor and even a cat was said to be under my chair! Any and all of these had to be painstakingly answered and explanations given, as to why in many cases nothing could be done about them, only for them to feature in different order and continue for as many hours as one can stand, before the sheer repetition gripped you and made you want to run screaming from the house.

Those several months of the year, from the Christmas through to Easter were a great toll on us both, although I have to say the condition allowed Mary to quickly forget, whereas I held the thought of it and over weeks it simply became an enduring mental torture. She was desperate that I didn't tell anyone in fear of us being parted, but as it continued night by night I knew I had to do something, or I just couldn't continue. Composing a list of the kind of questions and sightings of these people, who she could see when I couldn't, I addressed them to the doctor at the memory clinic. In truth it wasn't only medication that might ameliorate the situation that I wanted, but explanation if possible, for the visions did very much intrigue me.

Questioned about them I found they were seemingly stood, or seated, not moving and at times had been with me in the same chair. Not solid, but fairly substantial, yet faceless, although clearly male, female adult, or child. In particular their dress was modern and the colour of the clothing could be discerned, the first of these being a little girl in a bright blue dress. These 'visitors' would tell Mary things, such as I had gone into town, whilst she was briefly alone, when in fact I had only popped out to the garden and told her exactly what I was going to do and how long it would take.

A further aspect was that upon entering the room I'd be asked where John was, or the whereabouts of my brother and sister (I have neither!). My detailing this information in writing, was I found appreciated by the psychologist and subsequent to it being received, there was an addition and increase to medication; which for a while led to a much improved life. As the weeks turned to months, there of course were isolated incidents, but on the whole it would be true to say, that to a large part we got our lives back and it was wonderful while it lasted! However, we were still virtually house bound, for no longer could one tell what disruption might attend each day.

Confined to Barracks

Constant supervision though was essential, in the main in respect of the difficulty with mobility and sensory deprivation. Indeed there were days when as long as I kept on checking, say every half hour; an hour, or even two, could be spent outside in an endeavour to tame the gathering jungle that the garden had become. This area of household maintenance was necessarily much curtailed, for the relentless indoor necessities of cooking, washing and cleaning took the highest priority. After these were done along with shopping for the essentials, time had to be found for meeting calendar appointments. All with medical connotations for this and that, they often seemed to occupy two, or more days of any five weekdays.

We decided to try meals on wheels, but quickly discarded it, for these at best could be described as institutionalised and there is pleasure in cooking I find. Also well-cleared plates are likely, when fresh produce and fruit is combined with the best of meats and fish. Throughout this period I still pondered if it would be wise to attempt a short break of some kind, as opposed to the couple of hours or so driving around the local countryside; which although pleasant, were difficult to do without soon revisiting so many well-known places.

Indeed any thought of even a weekend break brought into play two important aspects for consideration, for in the first of these, might the change of location and absence of home environment, bring about an acceleration of the Alzheimer's, as had occurred at the move to hospital? Other than this the B&B would need to be disabled-friendly and at least have ground floor accommodation. In this respect the chance arrival of an 'Able' Magazine, provided better hope that one such might be located in comparison to the one visit I had been able to make to see what was on offer at a W H Smith store.

Easy Access Britain too, was duly purchased and found to have a wealth of information, however there was little of use to my particular need, for long distances could not be contemplated and there was a distinct lack of B&B locations within. I also purchased a RADAR key and their book of locations where it might be used. Once more it was well produced, but firstly I didn't want 99% of the listed locations and more importantly, a distinct absence of necessary, even vital information was exposed as not being within its pages. I will explain: Say you are in even a small town, not well-known, or even unknown and the book lists three, or four toilets by road name alone.

However, without some graphic notation, I find this of little assistance, for if someone is there and you can, or dare park to ask; from years of experience I know very well, that even locals rarely know any street names and little beyond their immediate 500 yards. What the book needs is even the most basic diagram within, say, a square inch or so, and a red spot to show where the toilet exists. This is essential and I say this knowing there are many even supposedly healthy and mobile persons who at times and for various reasons need this kind of information fast and as it is, I'm sorry, but in its present form this book too is of little use. The 'Able' Magazine however was, for within its pages there was much useful information, among which was a result in respect of the long unanswered question regarding the taking of a bath.

The purchase of a bath lift quickly put an end to this particular need and its so far reliable functioning was characterised perhaps best, by the prompt arrival of an engineer within a matter of days, to fit a modification that had been deemed necessary by its manufacturer. Sadly, this was however absent where the stair lift was concerned and as the months following its fitting passed, it was found to be most unreliable, stopping in mid-flight on numerous occasions for unknown reason and leaving itself stranded mid-way for best part of a week, but as I have already said yet more of this anon.

Further difficulty was experienced in regard to a wheelchair, which in line with the provision of other aids from the local authority had been efficient. This being so, the problem was that it was too heavy for me to lift in and out of the car, due to my having a damaged back of long standing and the rules for any replacement decreed that one must wait three months before anything could be done about it; well four actually, as I was later to find and this to me was absurd, when someone else could have been using it to full advantage.

This aside, like all other aforementioned aids of this nature that had been provided and once the time limit had expired, a swift and generous conclusion took place. We were invited to visit a supplier to ascertain if a lightweight chair to my liking was available, ahead of a voucher being issued. Once this was done, it was a simple matter of exchanging the voucher, which also covered maintenance of the chair and the former was then speedily collected for use elsewhere.

In actual fact the occurrence of this was delayed by a Christmas and year-end and an unwelcome increase in the Alzheimer's condition, once the dark evenings had returned. (It was in fact the type of Alzheimer's with Lewy bodies.) Thankfully, as I have said, there had been several months during which the prescription of both increased and an additional drug were no doubt the reason for an improved life style, but as the evening experiences were once more encountered, other factors would combine to increase my stress levels greatly. Some related to what might be termed as outside agencies, who obviously didn't know the aggravation they were causing.

Other than this quite a lot was related to the so called services for Carers and GPs who caused difficulty, possibly through their having too large a patient list, or their having insufficient support services. Government please take note, it's supposed to be the National Health Service and not the World Health Organisation! The latter aspect arose through commencement of a deterioration in my own health, coupled with things associated with Mary's general medical health. Nearly always it was something small procedure wise, unnecessary and irritating at any time, but the more so when it necessitated extra phone calls and visits to the surgery, let alone it also disrupted the work of specialists and doctors at the hospital.

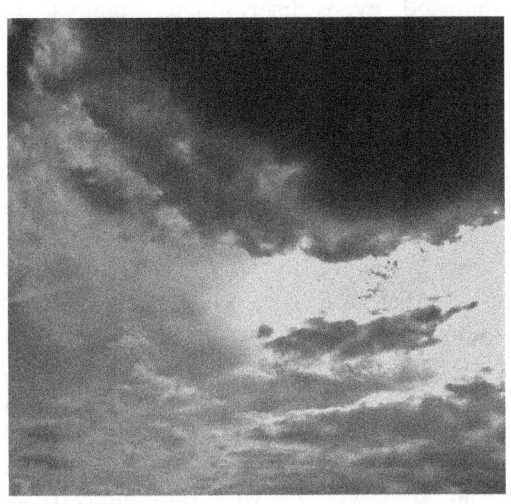

Respite ... it was not

Before such are explained more fully, it would perhaps be appropriate to state what respite from the caring role was ever offered, but more importantly how it was spent, for such explanation in my own case will rapidly expose it to have been of little help and of no particular consequence. Others may fare differently and good luck to them if that be so, but what would shortly be revealed, would lead to my feeling even more disenfranchised even discriminated against and for a variety of reasons.

Ahead of the two hospitalisations, an assessment had been made and following this a core time of three hours per week was commenced. It was carried out by a reliable and well-known organisation and so continued for a reasonable period, although it was in fact of greater benefit to Mary than I, in giving her female companionship and the chance to briefly get out to such as a place of interest, or to purchase clothes and cosmetics.

It, however, was not a sacrosanct three hours per week, for several things did curtail it. The replacement Carer obviously had two weeks holiday, around twice a year she was absent to attend meetings and on those occasions a replacement could not be guaranteed. Also during that first year I was prompted to ask Social Services, what would happen if I should be involved in an accident, or be taken ill while away from home during one of those times?

Was there provision of emergency cover, for my wife could no longer be left alone? Oh! we hadn't thought of that, was the response! My suggestion that something did need to be arranged, did prompt action and a contract to an organisation was awarded, but it turned out that it had no one spare at that time to be able to guarantee this. Advertisements were placed, but to this day my expectation is that the situation remains largely unresolved, for I was advised that on certain days I had better stay at home, therefore I had to be ready to take over at once, in the event of there being an emergency call out!

Thus of the fifty-two weeks of that year I actually got about forty-six and prospects for the following year were no better. Those few hours per week only allowed me to get my haircut, to take a bath, pop into town where I couldn't normally go, or have a couple of hours in the garden, but all were things that had to be done and therefore to my mind were not true respite at all from the caring role. All too often they coincided too with the need for me to accompany Mary to her hospital appointments, so in truth, although a break in routine, they had no therapeutic benefit.

For some ten or so weeks of the previous year there was also an entitlement covering a similar three hours per week from a different provider, but this was far from satisfactory for various reasons, thus the return of certain persons was declined and at no time did I choose to leave the sitter in sole charge of Mary. Thus those hours were used up working on the stairway, or working in the garden and house and likewise they did not give a complete break. In the event that by now you are wondering why I didn't choose to buy in help with the household chores, or garden, the answer has to be within the statement, "once bitten twice shy!"

Some recent contact with other Carers, quickly revealed that they had a general dislike of people for instance entering one's house at erratic times, to complete wash and dress routines. Not I hasten to say anything to do with the ladies we met in the six week post-hospitalisation period that this was carried out, but rather a seeming lack of co-ordination, or organisation through our learning they were directed back and forth across town and its environs, seemingly without any plan to best use these resources. This too, was evident where sitters were concerned, while a quick calculation that I made for that year showed that some ten respites were lost for one reason or another, possibly connected with the thirty or so hospital and similar medical appointments.

Having already stated my reasons not to take meals on wheels, some advertising led to me seeing a cleaning firm's van at a neighbours. Enquiring as to whether she would recommend them, I was to find she spoke highly of their fortnightly attendance, so I decided to give it a try. When the day came, there was no shortage of equipment unloaded from the van, so having earlier informed a supervisor of our needs, we naturally left them to it. A start was made in the bathroom by the two girls, but for what seemed forever, nothing except conversation was heard and no movement, or noise of vacuum cleaner came from the bedrooms.

An hour or so later the vacuum made a brief sweep of the stairs along with a quick soaking of the kitchen floor, then it was a rapid "Good-bye, see you next time". It clearly wasn't what had been promised and, apart from the kitchen floor being left with large puddles, a health and safety aspect if there ever was one, further examination revealed the accumulation of dust and dirt untouched elsewhere. The arrival of a bill for this pantomime prompted a call to the office and attendance of the supervisor, who soon found clear evidence for my complaint. The charge would be waived, while response to my saying I didn't wish to have another visit if this was to be expected, prompted her to beg that perhaps if I let her come with another girl, I might agree to the company's continued use.

No way I thought on the evidence to hand, for when I did it myself at least I knew it was done, even if a lot less frequently. Where the garden was concerned it was a similar story, but not because of laziness for this fellow was a hard worker and very punctual, but a little too keen if I could describe it thus. How? Well in early Spring, flower beds need removal of the dead growth along with weeds and leaving him to do this, my return was to almost bare earth. A day later this was explained when I lifted the lid of the garden refuse container prior to its collection by the council, to find many of my plants of up to 8 inch diameter, deposited within!

However this fellow meant well, so didn't suffer the same fate as the cleaning firm. I kept him, but made sure his arranged, but infrequent, visits were only for specific tasks where I was present and that association did continue for quite a while. In regard to other respite aspects along the way, and after no little encouragement, Mary did finally agree to attend a day centre on a one day a week basis. A second day was offered, but declined for reasons which need some explanation, for they in a large part are contributory to the lack of true respite that I complain of and were reason for the situation where I saw no end to an ongoing trauma and daily increase of doubt as to how much longer before I might have inability to cope with the task.

The Influence of an Unknown

To understand this I have with some difficulty, to go back to years before Mary and I met. Times of which I know little bar the smallest detail, but enough to understand that her thinking is based on a great deal of former unhappiness. Knowing and sensing that there was far more to this than was ever related, I made a point of not asking too many questions, but I think I gauge correctly that the failed marriage was perhaps the greater part, although latterly a further unhappy relationship was eventually revealed. There were too the salient times of bereavement and change of home that added to that and a somewhat chilling awareness that hate and belittlement somewhere along the way had likewise left deep scars.

At our first meeting, I quickly realised that she was very special and this was a feeling that received continual reinforcement during our two years of our going out together. Each of us had both separate and combined interests which could be shared and without great expense we could get comfort from the beauty and variety of the world around us. Of country stock, she had the down to earth goodness and simplicity, while embracing the sophistication of style, dress and fashion that made one proud to be seen with her at any time. Truth, honesty and reliability were inherent in her character and manifestly there was kindness, gentility and affection in abundance.

Mary too, had a great love of animals and especially so all babies and small children without exception, this latter aspect having the cruelly dealt blow of the loss of an infant, within an hour of its birth. From day one, we commenced the caring and sharing relationship that led to our deciding it should be ongoing and as traditionalists, believed this should be confirmed by marriage. Although by no means wanting in terms of general knowledge and the wider world, through reading and the enjoyment of her early years within family, teens and early womanhood, her chances of travelling further afield had been virtually non-existent.

This I resolved to change at the earliest opportunity and our early years together were characterised by the removal of anxiety in regard to stability of relationship, finance, security of dwelling and there was ample chance to explore and thereby discover not only Britain, but further afield in the pursuit of their countryside, history and heritage. If there is one word that might be used to express one's feelings about those years it is contentment. Without disagreement, without argument, a sharing of the tasks within the home and each of us having the opportunity to pursue the individual interests, along with those which we shared.

I know this sounds all too lovey dovey, but it is wholly fact and from it stems my own intense devotion to the newly arrived situation, however it also goes a long way in explaining the feelings of Mary herself, which today continually make the situation even harder. To an outsider, without compassion, they will be thought to be perhaps selfish, but I suggest one stops for a moment to review the background, which I can understand, even though it is not fully known. During our time together there has been continuity, security, love and understanding, which in many ways were so absent before.

What I have not stated as yet, is the death of Mary's father as she ended her teens. Is it not natural therefore that she has developed a deep seated love for all that I have come to mean to her, starved of love and affection to a large extent from that day on. She now only has myself, missing greatly in particular her mother, who then for short time was her only comfort and whom she misses so desperately. With memory now lost of all the years since, Mary believes her to be alive and each time she has to be told that is not so, it's as if she is being told for the very first time of its happening.

As if that wasn't enough, Mary is now forgetting almost everything as it happens, there is constant reminder night after night in the absolute terror of loneliness, not knowing where she is, why she is here and myself being the only constant in a world of emptiness. This being so any thought of our being separated, for even an hour, or two is anathema to her, even though she cannot now remember the marriage and often talks as if I am, but one of two persons. Taken to the day centre there were tears, tears too at any thought of parting, fear that I will not return for, like it or not, this dependence is both flattering and claustrophobic.

It had so far stopped any thought of my accepting a week's respite, for as good as that might have been for myself in particular, its effect upon Mary might have been to originate a further acceleration of the Alzheimer's, as happened so dramatically upon her admission to hospital. Our being so far down the road as it were at the time of meeting, we knew very much that the years together were limited and now after them being so good for us both. Neither of us wanted anything to restrict the chance of sharing whatever months, weeks, or days that were left.

It might have been like a noose around my neck at times, but I shared her devotion, for Mary was such a sweet dear soul and in some ways so good that one imagines she will have immediate entry to heaven one day, if indeed that place as we hope truly exists. This I emphasise is no adulation, no excess of emotion either, for 'Dear, sweet soul' has been a phrase stated by so many who have met her at shops, hospital, or wherever, through her smile, gentility and absence of even single attribute of any of the usual human defects.

All the more reason therefore to regret that this gentility is lost whenever the Alzheimer's cuts in, for not only does it replace a competent person with a lost soul, but totally eclipses the former who one knows and loves. It is I think best described, as an unpleasant entity that takes over. It's difficult to get one's head round this and I often ponder why and how this can happen. One assumes the change is within the brain, for it is described in print as being the result of a fatty gum forming at junction points, thereby stopping the accessing of information stored within the brain, but it in no way explains the fear and confusion which daily takes over.

Where the Lewy bodies are concerned I try to explain this to Mary, by saying it's like one's memory being a giant library, which now has barriers placed across its access paths, preventing one from getting to the books that hold those memories. Not exactly true in a couple of rare events, for last Autumn and again later she suddenly remembered her being called from home in the middle of the night to hospital (actually back in 1991). On arrival she was to spend her last few moments with her mother. That being so, she cannot now regularly remember and it is the reason for her compelling belief that she is still alive.

Returning to my point and that brief instance proves it. The memories are all in there, nothing is actually lost, it's just that they can't be reached. As such it is a reasonable proposition, but that's only the half of it, for the other things that happen are not so easily explained. Foremost of these is the feeling Mary often speaks of, located somewhere to the right of mid-body, she recognises it as the precursor of trouble and says it always appears ahead of the Alzheimer's cutting in. No item of the body thereabouts is presently known to act in such close conjunction with the head, so as to give rise to mental confusion, or have we yet to learn?

Likewise what I term as an entity, in appearing to take control, smacks of a biblical idea of being possessed by the devil, but how on earth can what is now known to be happening in the brain, produce this phenomena? Whatever it is, when 'it', this creature of the night takes over, it is all powerful, persistent in denial and refuses to accept anything other than 'it' believes, continuing long term as if taunting, goading, until it breaks you. There is certainly no credible explanation! So what about the soul within us too; yet another mystery!

Relentless Warfare

One cannot but wonder at the complexity of the human brain in its normal condition and as I have already indicated there is ready realisation of how the forgetfulness occurs, however, this aspect of a single purpose transformation into some kind of fiendish being is not only mysterious, but frightening! After more than two and a half hours, yet alone seven, or eleven, I challenge even the Pope himself to not submit and one feels so guilty that you cannot stay calm as you wish, but the constant repetition is pure torture and one knows not where to turn, or what to do and absolute desperation overcomes you.

I knew that I could not ask for help, much as I often wished, for it would split us, but having tried everything, nothing else remained except that we could head for bed. Only then did 'it' submit, peace of some kind returned and we could both pick up the pieces and start again as best we could next day. For my part such nights which were spread throughout two winters, took a heavy toll. Each is remembered as a scar on the relationship, which after 'it' (the vicious aspect of Alzheimer's) departed for a while. We continued as before, except that the normal confusion sometimes has amusing connotations. Unlike myself Mary remembers nothing, so is less scarred by those events.

The whole thing is cruel and devastating and as yet remains another scourge of today's world, which is already suffering cancer and various other vastly unpleasant things, all doggedly defying man's ability to master them. Often one's suspicion is that did we but know it, we ourselves are sowing the seeds of these modern ailments either in our manifold pollution of the planet, or the mass of chemicals today associated in various ways with food and drink production. Whoever the Carer is, be it husband, wife, child, or other relation in their charge, and whatever the cause of their requirement for service beyond the call of duty, the desire of each is to maintain and prolong the time that their loved one, or friend remains with them.

Hope springs eternal that some fresh treatment, or drug will be found to at least ameliorate their suffering and where this aspect is concerned I feel privileged that we have been supplied with certain drugs which to others one understands, are only available sometimes through great personal expense. This being so one takes each day at a time, all the time conscious of what is already lost, yet more often than not being able to feast on a few moments of shared happiness; laughter even arising from yet another snatch of conversation and weird remark that is emitted from God knows where and of no relevance to reality.

For example, a sudden awakening and being told "There's a dog in the bed!", or as of one night at half past midnight, "I want my umbrella!" Why? "I'll want it at breakfast." Other similarities included my being told there are two other men in the bed and her taking action to stop my supposed bleeding, from soaking the bedding. Oh yes and another too, that was related to bedding. Finding this being investigated along with her pyjama jacket, I enquired the reason and was told its texture was not unlike breakfast cereal and therefore its edibility was being considered! It's hard to understand what is really going on when such behaviour comes from anyone and even more so when it's someone who you love deeply and who for quite a large proportion of the time is still completely lucid, very sensible and rational in relation to thought, motivation and manual dexterity. True, more nodding off for periods of much more than forty winks was by that time more common and far less reading was taking place, although this was probably often more related to Mary's sensory deprivation.

By now, I think you will have gained a fairly good idea of the picture of what was going on within the four walls, from which there was so little escape without more external assistance. It could I know have been a lot worse, for as yet thank God we have yet to experience things like incontinence which may occur as the time passes and the prospect of much increased laundry load as a consequence was ever present. Some days were and are currently better than others, but even now I can detect changes in both the timing and nature of the disturbance to normality.

Over three nights for instance there were awakenings to remove curlers as a preliminary to a morning awaking, but they were at one and three thirty rather than at six o'clock. Could it have been the first signal that another aspect, that of losing touch with the internal clock which governs us day and night, was about to cease functioning? With this and other things constantly on the mind, there was enough to keep you on your toes and pretty well occupied, let alone coping with the daily routine of meal preparation and giving medication, which in themselves are quite substantive time wise.

Who ever said "A woman's work is never done" to my mind certainly hit the nail on the head. The needs of the outside world however need to be dealt with and it goes a lot further than just shopping. The days of local providers for energy and the like are sadly long gone, to be replaced with faceless bureaucracy and call centres who couldn't care a dog's leg about anything, other than getting home and out of their battery hen environment. Others may wish to spend what one gathers are hours on the phone pressing this and that and listening to un-wished for music, only at best to be promised things that never materialise, but that was not for me. Being old fashioned I still prefer to write, for proof exists of what is said and answer when received, leaves you with a positive response. Not anymore it doesn't, but I still try and have occasionally been rewarded by a reply from a like mind, but not that often!

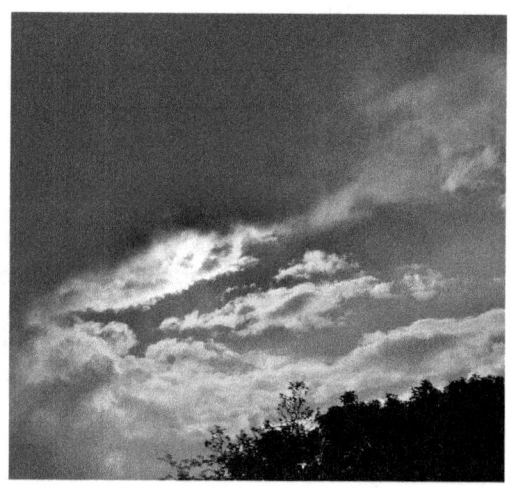

JOHN ENGLAND

External Aggravation

During those months it was one damn thing after the other where that kind of thing is concerned and it isn't reserved to public utilities and the like either. If anything the often much maligned British Gas comes up trumps, by giving special rates (that I didn't have to ask for), and unexpected cheques to help meet rising costs. So what aggravation could I recently have very much done without and who was responsible? For one take that stair lift. Twice during its first year calls were made for faults to be rectified. You couldn't ring every time it went wrong else you would be classed as a pest, so I kept a log so that the engineer would hopefully reach early conclusion of what was wrong.

After the first call I waited a week and while it was repaired asked that the track be tightened due to its extensive movement having been noted. At the second it was stuck fast half way and the week again being quoted I requested something sooner, to have it cut to four days. The chap this time seemed more proficient and upon leaving mentioned he had tightened the track. In fact both had, the first at the support bases, the second where the supports joined the rack. Joined up thinking, or what! Clearly a case of get out quick on the part of the first.

So far so good one might think, but it was only weeks when a letter arrived assuring me of the honour I must feel at having such a rare and precious commodity. Sheer flannel of course, to disguise the fact that year end approached and it was now time to take out a maintenance contract. Several and various hundreds of pounds were required for cover with, or without call out charges, or including parts, or not. Each of the lower amounts to be paid was deemed suspicious in that too many situations would not be fully covered and where electronic circuits are concerned almost every fault would require replacement of an expensive circuit board. So with little option it had to be the alternative, which was £1,500 full cover for three more years.

To my mind it wasn't as trading standards would say 'fit for purpose' anyway and I told them so, taking the opportunity to inform said Trading Standards of its performance to date. It did the trick and a couple of calls from that department ensured action that left it a great deal improved. Mind you it still has a hiccup every so often, but is far improved from what it was.

The local council was the next to spoil what till then had been a much appreciated arrangement where what I thought was a generous deduction (rebate) was made to former annual payments on the grounds of low income and disability. Six months earlier I had difficulty reconciling their interpretation of exact amount, when intermediate statements were issued, so I called at their offices expecting rapid solution. How could I be so wrong? Luckily there was a blue badge parking spot, but upon entry to the premises I was told "We don't deal with enquiries here, you must go to the town centre". Pointing out I couldn't get to the town centre, I was very reluctantly passed a phone to talk to someone upstairs.

He and I didn't agree, for to me they were saying that two and two equalled seven, or something like that, so sticking to my guns he had to come down to the counter; but without exactitude for what was said, I thought it absolute rubbish and we parted with the situation unresolved. Some months later when yet another statement arrived, firstly I did not understand why I had unearned income amounting to some £200 per week, or why Mary was said to have savings of almost 2K above what she actually had.

When a letter was sent in regard to this it took two not one before response and I was told they only took figures provided by the pensions people and the £200 was our combined pensions. I didn't bother to argue, but if like we you have paid in your National Insurance since 1946 and have worked full time, you don't consider the pension to be an unearned income, far from it. Before I pass on to the other thing I had asked about, there was one more surprise where the Council was concerned. I got a cheque in excess of £200 without any explanation.

Very nice on the face of it, but I read the warning about facing court proceedings if I wasn't entitled to it and I'm not the sort of person to accept an amount like that without wanting to know why, for I still had in excess of that to pay before financial year end! Need I say my letter was ignored, so in due course I completed the remaining monthly payments that were due and finally banked the cheque, in desperation of it ever making sense. With three, or four different addresses to choose from and related to pensions matters, it was a toss-up as to which was the most appropriate to write to, asking in relation to the supposed 2K, but suffice to say three went off in total, most unanswered.

Nevertheless, over time, I did get one which included the printed wording as follows - We understand you will shortly commence receiving your pension! My pension in fact started back in 1994-5 and with statements like that, is it any wonder the country is in such a mess! So much for officialdom, but it didn't end there for after a well appreciated deal from the NHS at local surgery level, things went haywire here also. Being tied as it were in not being free to go except I take my wife with me everywhere, I have chosen to drop my GP a letter, leaving him free to read it at his convenience and call me later if necessary. It seems it's no longer that simple. Several months back there was no reply over several weeks, prompting me to ring him direct.

"Hello", was the greeting, "How are you"? Somewhat surprised I said I imagined he would know, only to find he had never seen the letter that had been taken into reception and not posted. Helpful man that he is he said he would find out what had gone wrong and not only rang back, but visited and did all that was necessary on that occasion. Why had he not seen the letter? It had been filed away without him being made aware of it, despite being clearly marked in capital letters 'For the Attention of'.

A Revealing Insight

Where Mary's fate is concerned as an Alzheimer's sufferer one cannot apparently be specific, for everyone it seems is affected differently; however where this particular case is concerned and even if it might prove to be a little boring, I should provide some amount of detail in regard to how a mind can be affected and the weird resultant behaviour patterns experienced. Having mentioned, I am sure, the loss of some twenty years of memory some twelve months back, the tail end of 2009 brought further stress in that the happenings of only an hour or so previous were now lost.

To expand upon this theme I will now cite detail extracted from the information regularly passed to her consultant psychiatrist, in order for him to gauge how the path of deterioration was being witnessed. This daily and incessant repetition continued in respect of incidents on the fringe of the twenty year blanking out and related to the former home and the flat that followed it, with such as was a key left, or furniture and clothing? The motorised cycle is outside and has to be put away (sold 18 years ago). Her mother is alive! (died in 1991) and strongly disowns that her parents grave is maintained (by me) and questions as to the money for the flat being received?

Mary incessantly needs to return to mother who was left this morning and on other occasions this supposed old man who has been left in a wheelchair. People are now regularly seen within the house and there is fear that someone will come to get her and cause trouble. In late afternoon and throughout the evening hours there is a great fear and anxiety which relates to it being 'their' house, for we don't live here and the police will come, for it belongs to 'them' and she will go to prison. Darkness too is feared, so a light was kept burning on the landing throughout the hours of darkness, however this doesn't entirely relieve the situation.

Mary often talked about another house across the road that I supposedly own just like this one and when in the kitchen is surprised because I've got the same plants in this house as those within the supposed one nearby. It's bad enough if one mother long departed is still said to be very much alive, but the situation then becomes all the stranger, for it's a step-mother now too, that has to be seen as a matter of urgency and any amount of persuasion that this is pure fiction is rebuffed vigorously. Where our relationship is concerned, Mary often talks to me about John and it's as if there are two of us, where it is the correct detail of my previous work, etc, that is stated, as if it relates to the fictitious other being of her imagination.

Simply Unbelievable

Mary also now regularly spoke of a brother I certainly never had and when I said that without the addresses of people she wanted to visit, I couldn't take her to them, I was accused of holding her prisoner, that we were not married and she was only staying here, and is now married to another man, for we split up some time ago! Mary often said that her mother was here sitting in a chair earlier and insists she has a right to be taken to see both her parents and step-parents.

When I say it was not possible for her to have had a step-mother on the evidence I have, she even comes up with the name Whatling. It doesn't end there by any means for there are times when you are tempted to laugh at the sheer lunacy of the moment, so how's this for a sample? One morning after breakfast - When are we going home? We've got to get back to Russia! When are you going to this other house; 'they' will know all about 'this' and keeps on referring to the flat next door (when it's half of a pair of semi-detached houses).

It got even worse later, possibly as an effect of a Nuclear Medicine slug related to an over-active thyroid condition, for it was our baby's well-being that was the cause of concern. With the approach of Christmas 2008 there was further deterioration and from January 2009 the new nightly slant was that she must go home, for we were only friends, she likes me, but will marry 'him', presumably the other me spoken of so frequently. Next afternoon I was asked if he'd gone to his allotment with his shovel, so one can see the variations on the theme are endless. As a general rule it was only when I could get her to go to bed that some normality of behaviour returned, but as will be seen this was to become more difficult with the passage of time. Perhaps lying down increases the blood flow to the brain, I can only guess, but it's only around a third of the distance required when one is standing, or sitting up.

The real bonus (for the sufferer rather than the Carer), is that due to the memory loss aspect, nothing whatever is remembered, even amazing statements like I had murdered her mother, or called her a prostitute! These latter utterances were beyond belief and so totally out of character to our nature and former life of contentment together that they frighten still in their obscenity. Having related this general calm upon retiring for the night, there were however exceptions and one is reminded of the earlier history of being subject to nightmares.

In the early part of the night there could be calling out as she seemed to be wrestling with someone, or something and there was much head and arm movement. One January night was most peculiar for she growled like a dog for several minutes and when I endeavoured to waken her to break the dream, my finger was caught in her mouth and bitten, though not painfully. By February, six weeks of traumatic evenings had reduced me to being unable to concentrate, or do even the most simple task without constant interruption and argument.

It was clear that a change of medication and re assessment of her condition was imperative, otherwise we could not continue as we wished and remain together. One day, upon return around noon from a run into the country, there was continuous diatribe regarding it being imperative that she saw her grandmother, also a man that wants her to live with him, 'them' and a couple that want her to go into a house and up to bed. Also as ever she must get back, for her mother is waiting for her and all the usual demands follow, almost as if they were an orchestrated performance calculated to reduce the other person present (myself) to a nervous wreck. I certainly feel intense sadness to see Mary in this condition, it is so, so totally unlike the person that I know and love, so, so much.

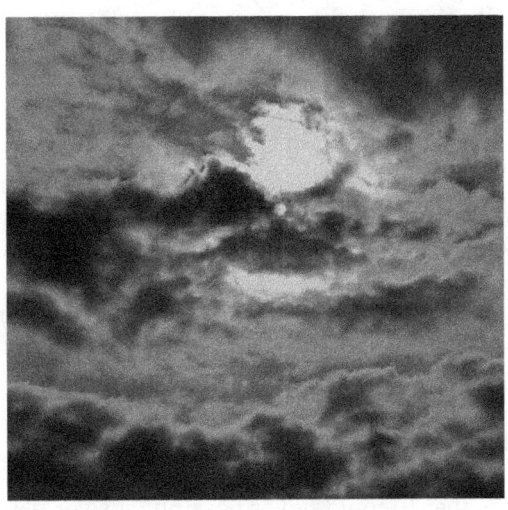

The Death of Communication

I too feel her confusion and disbelief if I tell her the things which she has said during these periods. It's especially difficult, due to my knowing that she fears something horrible and unknown throughout all these times. By now Mary was very restless, was unable to concentrate and the papers, or the magazines she loved were no longer read and it was the same with TV, Video and DVDs. Mary now became increasingly irritable, knew she was unwell, despaired of ever getting better and sometimes even said she wanted to die! To counter this I tried to ignore the past and concentrate instead on today and tomorrow. We both at this age have only limited time left together and this ongoing anguish for both of us is destroying our lives.

Day-time was often nigh on normal, except for forgetting to use the zimmer frame etc, but all evenings were traumatic and in particular those ever repeated demands that I could never possibly answer were taking a toll on me, despite understanding what is making them happen. In truth we are caught like rats in a trap, for there is no way out, it would only get worse with the passage of time, but I desperately wanted to hang on. It had been so easy back at the start to say that I would take it in my stride. I was sensible, I would adapt and could at no time ever think it would become too much for me to handle. How could I have been so wrong?

All very laudable, but that was then and this was now and the going was getting that much rougher week by week. If there was incontinence and physical work was needed it would certainly be tiring, but I was being sapped by what I termed never ending mind games. They drained me and the endless repetition was akin to that when the old style gramophone needle got stuck in the groove. Day after day there was no escape for me! Where confusion was concerned as an ongoing aspect, I provide here some further examples: I ask one evening what Mary is looking so intently at?

There was another cat under my chair! One morning she was looking at something, so I asked what it was? Some money was in her lap (Mary hasn't handled any money for eighteen months now). A regular at meal times was I've got some pills to take, when they've only just been taken and can't have even reached her stomach yet!

Other statements related to someone who is in the corner, or who has gone upstairs. Mary would ask, where were the people who had a meal with us, or that were with us earlier? She often couldn't picture our Tuesday relief Carer, my son, or even the hairdresser who had left us only half an hour earlier. She would ask where I slept last night, also were we married and where was her husband? Also when looking at a DVD music catalogue one day, Mary said there are some lovely holidays in here!

Some eight months later I now pick up the threads of my tale in an all too brief respite, following a week of pain and anguish. It is July 2010 and the previous two months have seen a rapid acceleration of the problem. No longer was it the evenings, but part and complete days of confusion and a point had been reached, where if something wasn't done I was going to go under and thus most likely put an end to my ability to stay with Mary in our home. The stair lift was still failing in mid-flight at least twice a week, council tax and other aspects remained generally unresolved, despite the intervention of a trouble shooter and almost all else was getting less and less attention, for I no longer had the energy, or inclination to bother any longer.

DARK CLOUDS HIDE THE SUN

That long and unusually cold winter of 2009-10 was now replaced by unrelenting heat and drought and its end should have brought a little relief from the Sundown Syndrome's peak at mid-winter. That certainly wasn't the case and the long past winter days were to reveal only increase in trauma for us both. Neither was there any amelioration brought about by a recent medication increase, as had been the case some twelve months earlier, for it was merely some concentration on the shuffling of timings, all of which were to no avail.

JOHN ENGLAND

Contact with Other Carers

During late spring and the commencement of the financial year, thought of the recently past months meant that I elected to postpone any take up of my allocated moneys till the autumn and the opportunity, to gain an extra three hours for seven weeks was taken up in order to attend a course entitled 'Caring with Confidence'. Originating with Leeds University as I believe, in conjunction with some Governmentally funded research. It was of course run locally with two instructors, with a well arranged programme of chapters to be covered and was attended by around fifteen Carers other than myself.

It rapidly became clear that the one reason that had brought forth these pupils, was the fact that in their various capacities, ages and caring roles, one and all had tried all they knew to cope, but could not say they had completely and thus wanted help. Some all too brief discussions with them in teams revealed their dealing with Alzheimer's, Bi-Polar, Parkinson's, stroke, etc, presented them with different and more physical problems to mine, but what I would term the daily mind games I was involved in, was quickly revealed to the tutors who readily deduced this in my body language. For each week's theme there was ample written material, but far too short a time for it to be covered. I also quickly decided it perhaps was of more use for those younger and inexperienced in life.

However, we three older men, whether from being in the trenches, or through involvement in trades and management, needed no ideas originating from behind a desk and those without the benefit of our much earlier and harder upbringings. For a case in point take stress, where such as bereavement can only be understood by those who have endured the loss and subsequent loneliness. Caring too has a great deal of stress, whether it be mental, or physical and there are times when you desperately want to run out screaming, or crack your head against a brick wall, but you just can't, however much you want to. I did at least agree the pause for deep breathing, even punching a pillow rather than the source of the stress, but the text book procedure was a load of pure and unadulterated b****cks!

Namely that one should stand tall, imagine it's a beautiful morning. You are out in the countryside, there's a blue sky, the sun is shining and you are stood beneath some fruit trees. They are apple trees, just look at the lovely rosy apples, let's reach up and touch one, why not pluck it and taste the juice! ... Well I certainly didn't buy that one and positively refused to participate in the charade by standing up and going through the motions. It was so patronising and where juice was concerned, let's say I felt it had already been extracted!

As I intimated earlier some Carers needed advice on handling money and where other aspects were concerned, the lack of knowledge about what help might be available was manifold. I found out too that I had previously been assessed, although not on a one-to-one basis as should have been the case and also that I apparently actually had a Social Worker, although subsequent experience leaves me wondering what good that has produced. Needless to say another assessment was to follow and carried out by phone, with the great disadvantage that being talked about in her presence upset Mary greatly. Do they teach them nothing, or are they just too thick to realise they are more hindrance than help, most of the time.

The real eye-opener though was learning how much was on offer for Carers to take part in. When emphasis was placed upon this, I noted one lady had a diary filled to the brim and could not find room for anything else, she even was as I understood attending a course at the local college. The fact that this could be astounded me, for my Tuesday's three hours had to end on the dot, for my replacement needed to leave promptly for elsewhere. Even where this course was concerned the replacement Carer from another organisation was under similar terms, thus on a couple of occasions I had to leave before the session had been completed.

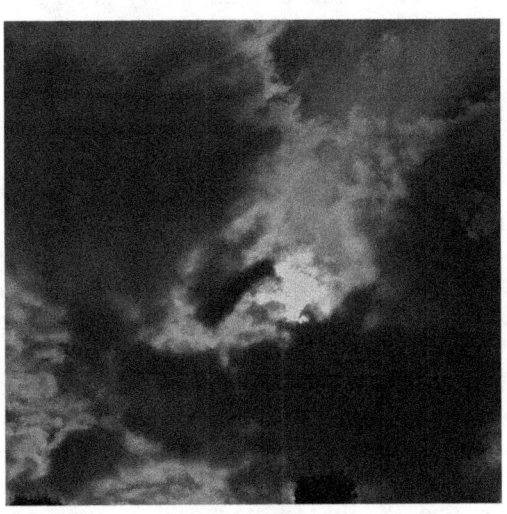

A Revelation

In that past two and a half years, as I have intimated earlier and without exception, the so called respite had been spent entirely involved with things that in no way were such a break. This insight into how the other half lived could not have become clearer one day, when it was mentioned that the facility had a very good cafe / kitchen and why therefore not adjourn there afterwards for a chat? When someone asked if they did meals, there was general decision to take up the offer and very nice too, but there was no way I could join them. So why was this and why were they not tied to a precise time?

The secret if that is the case, when it's more like the bleeding obvious, is that they all had friends and relations who were willing and able to help out. Where Mary and I were concerned these did not exist and totally in her case, for two long term friends in particular and years back, weren't even prepared to assist by walking with Mary 200 yards at most to a bus stop. For my part withdrawal from previous interests due to the caring commitment curtailed greatly what I could participate in. A year or more earlier, even the occasional Neighbourhood Watch meetings had to be forgone. Sadly too the world we grew up in and its values are now long gone and the mention of Alzheimer's itself is enough to clear the room, unless that is someone present, happens to have a relation so afflicted. The neighbours and those with whom she used to travel on the bus into town don't even ask anymore how she is; having one surmises, concluded that the matter is now closed and she is already consigned to the ultimate fate.

Confrontation and Aggression

That fate, did I but know it, was soon to take upon itself new and more acute manifestations, for as the weeks passed Mary's condition underwent substantial change and the task of caring was to become increasingly difficult and in the end wholly unbearable. It formed no particular pattern other than more of the same and was occasionally surprising, but day by day too, there was an increase in the measure of argument and for the first time aggression was to feature. In some ways I am loathe to cite more examples of the way the mind's confusion was manifested, for it is more a subject for the practitioner than those who are interested, in the light that being forewarned is forearmed; however I likewise feel it necessary to include this to enable some understanding of what can be encountered.

How about these as examples of what you can expect, all extracted again from information passed to the consultant. One morning saying 'thank you' to an imaginary man who has just gone out of the door, she suddenly said 'there's something here about low priced drinks' whilst looking at the floor, then talks about a mate she goes to see who has a little girl; all of these expressions conjured as it were from thin air. Asks in the early evening 'are we coming back here', then looks towards TV points to a nearby chair and says she is speaking to the Tuesday morning Carer, but it is Thursday and the time is 1020. 'Her husband is coming for her', (who!?) and then continues with 'I saw her looking through the window'.

DARK CLOUDS HIDE THE SUN

Waking on a Saturday morning Mary says 'you had better take me home' and will not accept this is her home, for I got her here through deception! 'Take me back, I didn't know, they didn't tell me, I can't stay here etc.' During one night she woke me around 0330 desperate to find a key, saying 'I've got to let mother in!'; also when retiring had asked what to do regarding a toilet as she stood beside the commode which had then been beside the bed for nearly two years! Constantly asking for me by name as if I'm someone else and not here with her.

During an evening a little girl was supposedly sitting by my feet, she is said to belong to the lady here earlier and when asked who actually came during the day and what she herself had done recently, has no idea whatever. For the second night in a week I am woken by her arms and legs flailing like wildfire (when she can hardly move during the day). I suppose it's another nightmare, but trying to wake her from it is nigh on impossible.

There too was a period with much sleeping during the day, in many ways a Godsend, however, upon each awakening there was an increase in the hallucination aspect and this in turn was followed by the commencement of serious accusations. All were demands to get back home, or to collect things supposedly left behind and were followed by statements such as 'you didn't tell me I was going to live here', with much emphasis on the fact that I had lied and deceived her etc.

Night after night this was to continue, with refusal to go to bed with me (a supposed stranger) without prolonged argument and provision of written proof of our marriage etc. Other aspects too arose that had not featured previously, regarding the fact that I was not administering her medication correctly and in particular the heart pills, also the police must be told that I was holding her prisoner, I was cruel and had struck her. I was keeping the whole thing a secret from her friends and everyone else too, inclusive of the weird thought that my religion and friends were reason for my behaviour.

Try if you can to visualise this situation, which commenced as a mainly evening time event lasting up to four, or more hours, but which now included the afternoon as well on an increasing number of days and ask yourself how might you cope with it? That question is very important as you will realise in time, for as my story proceeds, the incessant and never ending barrage of question, accusation and particularly the demands, wore me down as each hour passed and there was no escape from it whatever. I knew it would be the same tomorrow, the next day and the next, for within the time any response had left my lips it had been completely forgotten and the statements, questions, or demands continued ad infinitum.

Going back to the early days for a moment, of course I hadn't the faintest thought really of what it might be like later on, other than that it was likely that incontinence would normally feature. Knowing that little, I thus commenced this journey through hell and with hindsight, might it not have been better if I was warned of what to expect, but then with it regularly said that everyone's symptoms are different, I suppose this can hardly be predicted. I had certainly found this fact to be true in the few contacts made during the course for Carers and again much later also, upon attending a few meetings of a Carers group at the day centre.

In actual fact I think much of my particular difficulty lay in the diagnosis of Alzheimer's with Lewy bodies. Add to these fatty deposits that prevent access to memory, the instant memory loss and resulting confusion, anxiety, also the fear of something unknown and you have the sizeable problem I was facing day after day. Accelerated by the oft quoted 'sundown syndrome', as instigator of the ever more frequent outbursts, how was I expected to cope. Thus the bedlam of the mind continued taking its toll on myself, for my not having my wife's forgetfulness, this multitude of confusion steadily drained any opportunity for me to think clearly and complete what needed to be done. I found that I was forgetting to administer things like pills and eye drops at the correct times and on one occasion even missed taking Mary to one of her hospital appointments.

In general terms though I found I often had to go over the same ground twice as it were, when joined up thinking became increasingly difficult for me. This is an important thing at any time, but especially so for a Carer who has to live as it were the two lives and my experience of some work study routines many years earlier during National Service, had previously be found to be useful in this context, but not in fact any more. As of now, in one way or another, not only was one engaged in seemingly everlasting mind games, but also suffering psychical involvement.

Often being hit repeatedly during the night and told to get away doesn't do your self-esteem a lot of good, especially when I was doing everything you can for this person, neither did it help when you are woken to be told her father is in the top section of the airing cupboard! It now too became increasingly difficult to prepare meals, or even do the washing up because of constant interruption. At night there could be regular getting in and out of bed to collect clothing to take back to wherever and this related to a little boy she was supposedly looking after and who she must return to. It was a new twist on the having to get back somewhere for sure and where that was concerned it also required getting Mary back from the danger of falling down the stairway on several nights.

Throughout these weeks changes to the timing of administering medication were experimented with and so little advantage gained that in some desperation, I asked might I not have some sedative, or other in order to calm the situation. When none was suggested I rapidly concluded that as far as pills were concerned there were none any stronger that could be given and things were rapidly coming to a head. Indeed that was no understatement, for another aspect was that on numerous times the mumbling of unintelligible sounds rather than words were heard and statements and snatches of conversation were often far removed from reality.

On hearing a noise while washing up I went to investigate. I was to find her searching for her curlers and talking to a man supposedly sitting in my chair, who was helping her look for them. He was described as middle-aged, and wearing grey trousers and a blue jacket (this detail amazes me from a so troubled and confused mind). Later on I was told that a different man has been sitting on the sofa and she said that a book has been put on her lap! Having finally managed to get her to accept the idea that we go to bed, around midnight I was woken by her calling out and I am punched in the back once more.

This of course was not unusual due to bouts of vivid dreaming, but unlike previous occasions when she has been wakened with difficulty, this time I found it impossible for more than ten or so minutes. I tried shaking her hands, nudging her, tweaking her nose and shaking her more vigorously while calling her name, but all to no effect. Instead there was grunting, moaning, a fusillade of flailing arms and legs, screaming out and a torrent of unintelligible and anguished animal sounds, while her body convulsed. These latter movements had been seen and felt before and were quicker than can be counted; all from a person who has great difficulty in moving without dizziness!

It was certainly very disturbing and I was left wondering could it be a fit of some kind, but it would not to be the last as you will learn. Where aspects of her associated eyesight problem was concerned, several lengthy attempts were made during this period by the hospital to gain some improvement to the double and treble vision Mary experienced, plus the reported clouded sight at variable times. For the former the fitting of prisms would normally be possible and the latter might be eased through laser treatment to the back of the eye, however, neither were successful, it being stated that the eyes themselves were good and the fault lay in out of sync messages within the brain.

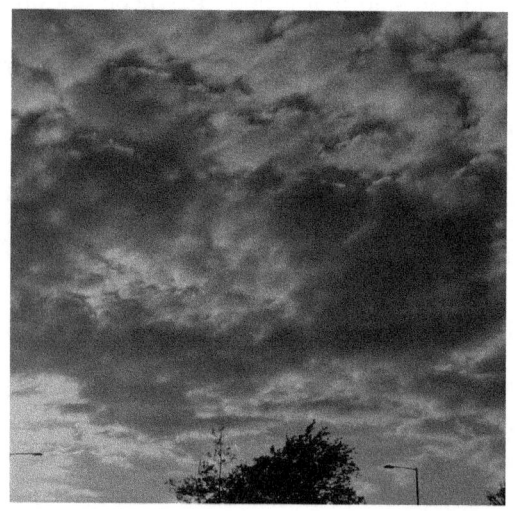

Complication of wider issues

Something very strange was certainly going on within it, for a further incident one evening brought the first involvement of a neighbour with my difficulties. For once I had actually been able to watch the TV news and a DVD while she had drifted off to sleep and thus been given a period of respite from her world of confusion. Such periods were certainly scarce, but very welcome and having this time lasted for a considerable period, I now deemed it appropriate to awaken Mary, for I was intrigued by a variety of facial contortions and other bodily movements.

However, in a similar vein to the night occasion mentioned earlier, any attempt proved to be impossible and I began to seriously wonder what might be the cause. After around fifteen minutes it looked to be serious and I reached for the phone to seek advice from a former nurse living nearby. Explaining the situation, she immediately offered to visit and advise, for no way did I want to ring for an ambulance, or doctor and have any admission, however brief, precipitate a worsening of the Alzheimer's condition as had happened before.

At this lady's arrival she found things as I had described and neither could she at first change it. At long last there was a fleeting sign of life and then it was back to lifelessness and her advice was to call for assistance. This done a promised call back fortunately came while she remained with us and gave her the opportunity to better describe to the controller the background and need to avoid a hospital visit. Success! A visit from a doctor would follow about an hour later. What did he find you might ask? A totally normal individual, laughing and joking as if nothing had happened; I felt a proper idiot I'll tell you, but he was very understanding and, after carrying out some basic checks, said I had done the right thing and he strongly sympathised with the view, that Mary should if at all possible be kept away from hospital.

It's nice to find doctors and their like agreeing with you on occasion, for the life of a Carer is a lonely one. You don't get out to see people that often and feel in many ways cut off from the real world, although the way it was going and what could be seen and heard of often made me wonder where it will all end. It's so far removed from the world of the 1930s that I grew up in and has lost rather than gained value, despite the many achievements of science. Right, that said as a further reflection on today's world, back to the doctors statement and in fact this was the second such in a matter of weeks, for another had said similarly at a routine thyroid clinic attendance, where the dizziness and movement difficulties had been discussed.

This dizziness of course isn't confirmed when positional hypertension tests are carried out, so again it may well be a matter of eyesight and message sending and if so this too, was getting much worse. Enough that is for me to request a home visit from the doctor for both it and the increasing difficulty of movement. This took place one evening and again I was left feeling I wished I'd never asked, for the blood pressure tests by a lady doctor showed nothing abnormal. By now I knew of course, that the patients view on things was sacrosanct and where this was concerned that one was, but a bystander.

So didn't that fellow Murphy have a heyday! Dizziness? - I never have any problem with it and I can move around all right when I want to! As if to confirm it subconsciously, a visit to the kitchen was made without the slightest difficulty, leading the doctor to say rather pointedly, 'I don't see any problem there, she did that all very straight-forwardly!' This was the problem that I had all the time, for other people didn't see what I saw, or for that matter have any comprehension of what trauma now existed on a daily basis. Whether it be the relief Carer, a chance, or infrequent visitor, even doctor; none when they visited would think there was anything wrong at all!

All those details provided to the consultant too, read like a fairy tale, but at least he understood, for the reason he was pleased to receive fairly regular updates from me was that the information was for a case study he was compiling. This is very understandable for I now gather that Alzheimer's with Lewy bodies, denotes a less common version of this harrowing complaint! That being the case, or not, it's very noticeable increase since April was by now gathering ground and the number of early afternoon through to evening periods was up to as many as four out of five.

There was great restlessness and the anxiety factor took such a hold of Mary now, that and the associated insistent and unrelenting questions and demands for the impossible were driving me crazy. Hour after hour they continued regarding her mother, father, house, flat, clothes, furniture, keys, money and all else long passed that she imagined was instead relative to the present and thus had to be dealt with immediately. The fact that it could not, only aggravated the situation more and this theme of I'm being kept prisoner, they don't know I'm here and you'll have to get someone in to sort it all out, was thus heard both longer and stronger. There too, wasn't a snowball's chance in hell of getting anything done either now, even the essentials, for this obsession to everlastingly keep on and on was slowly, but surely breaking me.

It too was not only when at home, for I had normally aimed to have a couple of hours driving around out in the countryside every week or ten days. This was a treat that Mary had loved so much in past times, but it now became far less frequent, for there was no hope of concentrating on the task of driving safely with a barrage of staccato sound in your left ear. Another previous delight had been a run out to a particularly fine hostelry for a delightful meal of traditional fare every couple of weeks or so, but this too had to be abandoned after the last such visit was marred midway, by a similar outpouring which caused me embarrassment in front of others present, that were within easy earshot.

Nothing it seemed could stop Mary's mind from doing a sudden change from normality to downright absurdity. TV, DVDs, video, books, magazines, music, history all had ceased to give interest and now it had become solely this obsession that occupied her thoughts. Although she often spoke of me to me as if I was someone else. I too as the person with her continually became the object of her troubles. I was responsible and the proportion of waking time when things could be said to be near normal and a loving relationship existed, had now dropped from 70%, to I would guess around 20% at best. At the back of my mind I knew it couldn't continue this way, but what could I do?

When it gets to a point when you have to turn off the kettle four times due to interruptions, when you are simply trying to make a cup of tea it is really bad and that wasn't the all of it by far. There was no way out though and I suppose, in some kind of desperation, you subconsciously eternally hope it will get better, but it never does. It most certainly got worse, until the near neighbour with hearing aid, or not, must have heard the heated exchanges when there was no way I could do as she insisted and repeatedly call the police, for dementia is not one of their priorities. This being so, I must confess that on other occasions I did threaten to, hoping it might quieten her. Likewise saying I would call a doctor and instilling the thought that this might result in her being taken away, was another vain attempt to stop the flow and calm the situation; but in truth only getting her up to bed was a 90% solution, if only that could be done.

JOHN ENGLAND

Crisis Point is Reached

Try as hard as I could to convince Mary, she insisted I wasn't her husband and she nightly refused to go to bed until persuasion was exhausted and the riot act had to be read to promote action. Until now there had been good chance that within an hour of retiring she would revert to normal, however that phase ended and the mornings now often began with guilt for having stayed overnight, what would her mother say! Increased too was the confusion as to where she was, mostly the streets of another town were transposed in her mind as being at a nearby junction and their houses were across the road. Many were the times I had to take her to the window to show her where she really was and explain that so and so didn't live next door and never had.

This increase in her total confusion was really getting to me, for a chance weighing of myself revealed I had now lost over a stone in weight, had too commenced wetting myself due to the emotional strain and was increasingly losing my grip on life. What though could be done, for there was no way I wanted my wife to be taken into the local hospital's mental ward, which I had had sight and sound of one evening years back, while delivering a letter to her psychiatrist. Any giving in on my part would not only betray the vow of 'in sickness and in health' made some fifteen years earlier, but likewise I might face her condemnation for putting her away; when during those same years I had done absolutely everything I could to make Mary's life different and wholly worthwhile.

Nevertheless day by day the signs were there that I was fighting a losing battle, unless that is a further change in medication might save the day. After a fortnight of increasing problems I, therefore, seized the opportunity to contact the mental health nurse while my wife attended the once weekly day centre. That fellow Murphy again intervened, she was not available, but I was promised that the consultant would ring me later. This he did, but could offer nothing new and merely suggested yet another alteration of pill timings.

I complied readily hoping against hope, however, from when Mary returned home there was no discernible change and I virtually had no sleep during the following nights. When the weekly substitute Carer arrived on Tuesday morning for her three hour stint, I naturally advised her of the situation, prompting her to call her control as she departed and say they should advise Social Services that I could no longer cope. This done, I felt it right to seize the opportunity to write to my doctor to this effect, with copies for my wife's doctor, her consultant and my so called social worker.

Those to the consultant and social worker went by that day's post, however, no response to the care agency message was received throughout the next day, Wednesday! Also early on Thursday morning the letters to Mary's and my own doctor were handed in to the surgery desk, yet note that from that time on to Saturday afternoon, no response was received to any of those four letters!

Notwithstanding this, as of Thursday lunch time, there was a further escalation and Mary became dramatically worse, till during the early evening I could stand it no longer and rang the emergency number displayed on the card I had always carried in my wallet. Its real purpose, of course, was for use if by any chance I was rendered 'hors de combat', by illness, or accident during those all too brief hours I was off the hook, but now there was an emergency and I desperately needed someone to take over for a couple of hours, in order that I could get my senses in order.

The result of the call? Several minutes of classical music. When it ended and a person finally answered, one had to provide such a host of detail that by then I was wondering why an earth had I bothered, for this conversation simply revealed my supposition of standby cover being available was pure fallacy. Maybe in an emergency perhaps, but I was very much alive and not ill, so I must wait for someone to ring me back.

That wait was possibly of twenty minutes to a half hour, when there began a lengthy conversation reminding me much of what I had once been told about by a person who applied to join the Samaritans. They had soon decided not to pursue their enquiry further, on learning that you didn't need to answer problems with advice as such, but just keep the caller talking till the heat goes off and, therefore, one supposed, ensure a fee was earned from the phone company for keeping the line in use? Anyway I was told an assessment would be made, however, when this would be made was not revealed.

Oh yes and what gem did I receive from this person on the other end of the line as their solution? 'Put the television on and let your wife watch the tennis!' Priceless! and it immediately classed her as obviously a fellow member of the 'juice extracting' fellowship, that came up with the 'let's reach up for these lovely apples', some months earlier. This call would also reveal something else that didn't exist which most certainly should have done. - It was that no record apparently existed of the Tuesday call to Social Services from the relief care provider, and nor was there any record of my several recent letters to my only recently discovered social worker.

It all supported my somewhat jaundiced view of the help for Carers in general being somewhat pathetic and there were to be further examples too, later on. So that was it, I was really no further forward after the effort, only in respect of knowing that this assessment would now take place. With still no response to the four letters by the next day Friday, its afternoon did, however, bring yet another long phone call (the assessment) and suggestion of a further day care opportunity, even though I had been told recently that no such vacancies existed!

Likewise there was an offer for a washing and dressing routine to be instituted, supposedly to help. This I turned down immediately as impractical, for with the arrival times for such spanning around three hours twice daily, it could only add more disruption and solve nothing. By 0830 on Saturday the situation was again bad, with no outlook of it improving and again I was forced to ring for a neighbour's help in calming the disturbance.

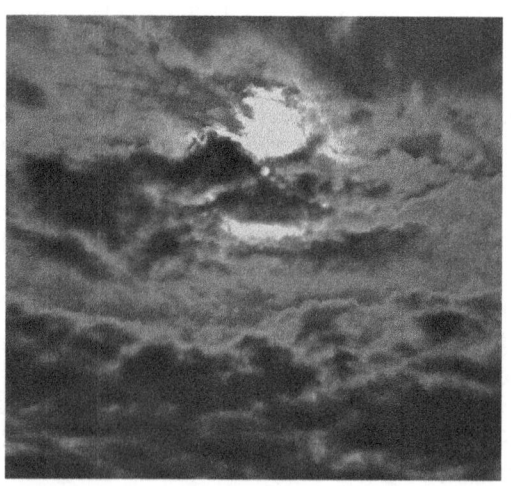

An Air of Finality

This was achieved but temporarily and within an hour Mary again became aggressive and commenced screaming at high volume. In desperation I called him back to the house, although I'd rather have bitten my tongue off and this time it was again to answer her demands to get someone in to tell her who I was and then presumably take the actions that were being denied by myself. This gentleman was a retired civil servant and like the former nurse had the understanding which comes from having endured such behaviour from one of their own relatives and two such where he was concerned.

His approach was to follow the recommended agreement with requests as a matter of appeasement, in the hope that what is demanded will be quickly forgotten and sure enough it worked fairly well with his even offering to take her thence in his car, if she could tell him the address. Of course she couldn't remember, so in due course he departed and I was left feeling that perhaps the text book approach was right after all, for something close to normality returned for a short while. Indeed it might have been an hour or so, but no longer, for during the whole afternoon it was I she berated, as to why he had not done as he promised. This and later instances lead me to think that when you are in an impossible situation it's better to stick to the facts, for any lies white, or otherwise and any untruth, will only lead to eventual exposure.

I'll grant you this, it's certainly a quick fix when it's a comparative stranger that does it and there remains an air of being of better behaviour when they are around, but if it's only a loved one that's present there are no such restraints and you receive full measure. This gentleman's wife later rang to say they had talked my situation over and decided to call the out of hours doctor service, in the hope that he might agree to a sedative being administered, however, at this time there was an inability to get the call accepted due to busy lines.

They having tried again later I was then told a doctor would attend, but a nurse then rang instead to reveal that she was expecting myself to be the one in need of the doctor! That confusion ended, I was told that a wait of four to six hours could elapse for this was non urgent treatment! This agreed (what choice had I), it was around 2030 when a doctor arrived and, after making basic checks of my wife's chest, temperature and urine announced that there was nothing wrong with her!

This decision as you might guess being vigorously supported by Mary. However, when her awe of his presence subsided for a moment, she commented that she wouldn't be coming so often in future, prompting him to enquire what was she talking about? When it was explained that she was convinced she had only come to see her friend (myself John) and would shortly be returning home to her mother, his response to me was. Ah! Yes Alzheimer's - you should understand this does vary from day to day and there is no cure; so you should get used to the fact! The patient is clearly OK and in the circumstances, any administering of sedatives was inappropriate!

His arrogance, the ignorance and the insensitivity for a moment stunned me and I would have received no greater shock in that moment if he had kicked me in the groin. I could, of course, responded to his puerile comments vigorously, but contented myself instead by biting my lip. He had no idea at all what it was like being condemned to being locked away hour after hour without respite and as such, his being called on my behalf with much good intention, had proved to be a thoroughly worthless exercise! Early next morning it was the next door neighbour who Mary demanded must be summoned to explain who I was, after photos, my bus pass and the envelopes of letters had been presented in the hope of settling this oft asked question once again.

In fact it was his second visit within a couple of days, for he had earlier answered my request to try to get her to stand up after I had endeavoured to help her, only to have her to fall back several times into her armchair. Complaining as she often did of just not having the strength any more, my thoughts now centred around the possibility that this was due to messages not getting through to enable muscles to respond to commands. This I was never able to determine with any satisfaction for events were now drawing ever more rapidly to the point of no return. Much as I wanted to as it were weather the storm, I knew I was virtually beaten.

The inability to get my head round things bothered me greatly, for I had always mastered situations and abdication wasn't ever a considered option. After nigh on eighteen months without Mary having a fall, these too now suffered a recurrence to complicate matters the more, plus she was now getting so anxious and overwrought that the long dormant chest pain and palpitation problem had resurfaced as an almost daily occurrence. One of these new falls was more easily described as her slumping down in the kitchen and there was no way I could lift her.

The neighbours had been bothered far too much of late so there was no way I could contemplate calling for their help again, the only thing I could do was drag her to the bottom of the stairs. Once there, there was opportunity for me to ease her onto the footrest of the stair lift as a means of slowly lifting her to a point from which she could gain an upright position.

This action had solved the problem on previous occasions, but the next fall would happen away from home on the following Monday morning as we arrived at the day centre and benefit to a degree, from the second of the series of Carer's meetings which had been recently instituted at that location. It was in fact another of the places where my body language rather than speech alone, gave ready realisation of the strain I was now under and its organiser was to become a welcome instigator of actions that would aid me greatly in the short term, although bring great sadness and trauma in the longer.

True I had already cried for help, thus already crossing the line that might cause Mary to blame me for what was inevitably to happen did she but know it at some time in the future, but even having made that phone call and written to the doctors; I desperately needed for it to be someone else who made that ultimate decision. One thing though had happened and this was a decision that I should now have a definite period of respite, although my wife did not yet know it and a preliminary a visit in preparation for those two weeks was to be made during the following week.

To all accounts it seemed a nice location and with no exact idea of where it was, I decided to use a trip out over the weekend to reconnoitre its whereabouts. Not an easy task as it happened and a deal of changes of direction and our finishing up in a dead-ended car park instead, sadly gave the game away as to what was afoot. I now well and truly had my work cut out for any separation, even while at the day centre, was cause of tears and it would be an uphill task to encourage her to accept being away from me for as long as a fortnight! We now approached another weekend, that alone guaranteeing that things would get worse and those two days culminated with a night of total rebellion.

When it was time for bed she would not take her tablets, declined to even put her hair in curlers and refused point blank to go upstairs to bed. I pleaded and begged without success, so there was nothing for it but for Mary to sleep on the settee and myself to lie on the floor. It had to be the floor, for when a down stair armchair, or indeed a garden chair taken upstairs was used following her hip operation, both were I found most uncomfortable. More than angry that it should come to this I was not pleased and hindsight reveals that a further prophetic statement was made in the heat of the moment.

Hoping above hope that I might change her mind in that last moment I said - 'If I have to sleep on the floor, I'll tell you now it will be the last night you sleep in this house!' Come Monday, the journey made across town for the 0900 start was completed with some difficulty, with Mary then moving the 30 feet or so to the doorway with the aid of the wheeled walker. As often was the case the eyesight determined that the door frame was hit and seconds later she herself slumped to the ground.

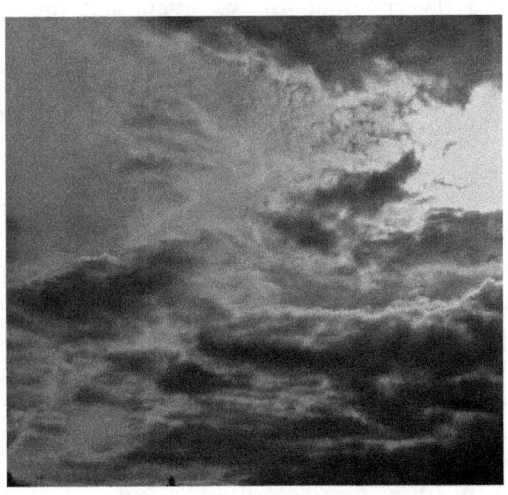

The Death of Separation

Sufficient to say the day centre dialled 999 and in remarkably quick time a paramedic arrived. By this time of course Mary had regained consciousness and with nothing broken it would seem, his prognosis was that she should return home and await the arrival of a doctor sometime later. So near and yet so far, I thought, and prepared to thus again lose my expected four or so hours of respite. More particularly though I was no further forward and the outcome of the event left me with an uncharged situation.

Not quite so in fact, for the day care supervisor, being well aware of what I had been enduring had, unknown to myself, already decided to advise Social Services, so action was in fact already being taken. First readied for a return home, then told to wait, then asked to return inside, we were in limbo for possibly an hour, or more, before I was summoned to the phone to receive instructions. My wife must remain, I was to say nothing and return home immediately to pack a bag and await its collection.

This having been done, the driver was to pick up Mary and transfer her to the respite centre in a nearby town which had already been designated to take her for two weeks in little over a fortnight's time. I meanwhile must see a doctor, who it would turn out want an ECG and insist that my health and well-being take first place, until such time as I was suitably rested, built-up and restored. Easier said than done in the circumstances, but difficult, or not it had to be done, for I knew if I didn't take heed I was heading for serious illness. Thankfully the ECG reading was OK, as were the other tests, but his offer of tablets to reduce stress was declined.

Within around a week I had a second appointment, at which the 'medicine' prescribed was rest and to occupy myself with long neglected interests for their therapeutic effect. Any thought of taking a holiday was out of the question, for I remained too concerned of what the sudden change might do to Mary's condition. I had no alternative though but to agree to give it a day or two before visiting her, however, I was more than apprehensive and totally lost without her by my side. It was one thing to pray for some relief from the trauma, but when the storm subsided I felt like a fish out of water and so desperately alone.

Now a Minor Miracle

Expecting the worst in regard to the effects of a sudden move and what effect it might have on Mary when I ventured out into the country to see her, I would indeed receive a shock, but not the one I expected. Instead of her being worse, I was to find her with much puzzlement as to what she was doing in this place, but other than this to my total amazement, sweetness and light had taken over and rather than the nightmare that had me as the villain, I was suddenly, as they say, flavour of the month, or the best thing since sliced bread!

That 'Honeymoon' lasted over two weeks and God was it good to be back where we used to be, gentle, sensible, loving, holding hands, kissing and cuddling, to once more enjoy the contentment that had symbolised our meeting and the marriage that followed. Was this all too true I pondered, because it was far from what had been expected by any means; so what had caused it? I had to know and the best way was to seek advice from her Consultant.

Another aspect that intrigued me, were aspects of the new care provision, for, due to the suddenness of the event, no introductory visit prior to admission had taken place. I found it difficult for instance to accept that after following precisely the directions of the Consultant in respect of timing, pill distribution was now more in terms of twice a day. His response was to advise with a most kindly nature that the remarkable change in behaviour pattern although perhaps unexpected, was not unknown after a change in both environment and Carer.

Some Misgivings Emerge

More particularly he went on to say this respite would go a long way in enabling me to continue to support Mary at home if further periods of respite were taken and his hope was that this situation would continue when she returned home. I would ask that you remember those words, for they were in print and those of her Consultant, who one would think above all would be the person who might best judge the situation, however, as will now be seen, this most certainly not the case. Still thinking at that stage that Mary would only be at that location until a more permanent place was found nearer to home and without the eighteen mile journey out to it, I accepted readily that it was a well-designed and modern site.

It was also scrupulously clean, the food was excellent and it appeared at first to be pretty well organised in its routines. This being so, as the days went by this view changed somewhat in that small things ruined the overall picture and spoilt it most unnecessarily. For a start although laundry was included, I said I would take care of it, primarily in regard to not wanting to lose items, but despite a large notice being put up to this effect they kept disappearing and mostly after only one day's wear. I arranged that she should have a daily newspaper, however, this stopped almost immediately and it was only after around three days that someone could tell me why; namely the newsagent had cancelled it through confusion with another resident's departure.

Where medication was concerned there were other rules too that made very little sense to me, even though I admit a lot of my problem was finding it more than difficult, to let go of the caring role I had had so long. For instance a Nitrolingual spray that was supposed to be taken when required and likewise Gaviscon, could not kept in the room, but specifically asked for (if only of course Mary could remember!). It was even more complicated in respect of a low dose antibiotic, where an extra tablet was only occasionally required and a long-standing arrangement was in place with her GP that I might give to a maximum of three.

Now, when urgently required one afternoon, difficulty arose because this doctor's agreement with myself was of course not mentioned on the box's label. My explanation could not be accepted, so a local doctor had to be consulted before the pill, could eventually be given several hours later! All of little help when the patient was in pain and discomfort. More importantly though, without that planned introduction due to the emergency admission, I didn't know what was available, my way around, the correct procedures, the intercom system, security alarms, or who was who among the various members of staff, for although I had since seen that identity tags were to be worn, they were in fact wholly absent.

JOHN ENGLAND

Unpleasant Encounters

Some weeks into this new lifestyle of infrequent travel by car due to the expense factor, versus time-consuming journeys through country lanes using my free bus pass, my joy at again having a loving wife eager to see me almost every day, was shattered by the face of officialdom. That which had been for so long unhelpful and uncaring, was now unduly anxious to jump in with both feet of its own volition and, contrary to any view as expressed so kindly in the communication I had received only days previously from the Consultant, it was distinctly abrasive.

It was to come in the shape of two females who interrupted our conversation one afternoon, requesting that I leave the room. They had to talk to my wife alone and it transpired it was not the first such assessment they had conducted and after this it was my turn to be interviewed. The words Starsi and Gestapo spring to mind and, through it all, I was acutely conscious that I had somehow committed the ultimate crime, in writing that letter to my doctor. It had started the wheels turning and like it or not, once started they would grind their way seemingly without regard to feelings and hurt that would result over the weeks and months that lay ahead.

To say it was a bombshell would not be any exaggeration, but more than this, it brought further pain in that from that time on, I began to experience doubt as to whether what Mary now told me was true, or part of some emotional blackmail linked to her Alzheimer's condition. Along with a load of gobbledygook she had apparently told them, its underlying theme revealed that she was accepting being incarcerated and had no complaints. Indeed there was some proof in that she apparently now bathed and showered when required, after refusing point blank to do so week after week while at home.

What Mary repeatedly told me, however, at each visit was very different, she didn't want to be there, wanted desperately to come home and was tearful at every visit upon my leaving her. Because her memory was now virtually non-existent, I had been jotting down which days she could expect to see me and including words of endearment to ease the pain of separation, such as the fact that she was never out of my thoughts and that I loved her dearly.

This must stop at once I was told! It was unsettling her and was stopping her settling into the new existence. The new buzz word was self-empowerment, so not only must I not see her so often, but neither must I help her while she was eating (despite her eyesight problem). Thus ironically all notes were now forbidden, but in contrast I could add information about visits to the calendar, and if that isn't ridiculous double speak I don't know what is!

So much for caring, I thought, more like domination and so, so callous, as if it was a thing, not flesh and blood, which such instruction related to. Did these people come from another world with their ideas that were so foreign to we of another age? It hurt a lot I'll tell you, for our meeting had been late in life and we had both greatly enjoyed these recent years, were desperate for them to continue and remain together, not only through life, but afterwards too, where internment was concerned. After thinking long and hard, I did concede that 'one-to-one' care couldn't continue once out of the home, but the harsh reality of this moment was more than difficult to stomach.

At my second encounter with the 'Stasi', I felt that I perhaps faired a little better, after producing the letter I had received from the Consultant and sticking to my guns, whilst concentrating on the importance of us having time together while we could. This I insisted should bear in mind our age and that the present improvement was certainly not likely to last. Only days later there was to be another unexpected arrival, thankfully by a far more acceptable person, who also revealed that she too had already made visits to Mary in the manner of an assessment. Having done so she now wished to talk with me, however, convinced we were talking about her, Mary became disturbed, followed us out of the room and constantly interrupted any serious conversation.

This person advised me that she represented an Advocacy service which was co-opted by Social Services and she would be seeing me several days later at a 'Best Decisions' meeting, which would be deciding the way forward. Of course I already knew the way forward and had long dreaded the time of its arrival and, in my innocence, expected that such a time might be delivered with care and sympathy akin to that one would expect to accompany bereavement. Not so by any means! For, even though its happening would signify the end of life in each other's company, it was very formal and certainly most intimidating, lasting for somewhere around two hours.

My hope was that the Consultant might have been present and that some discussion might therefore be possible, however, unfortunately he was not and my feeling throughout was that the several women officials had already determined the outcome and I was already judged as guilty of some heinous crime. The letter to my doctor received further mention and, if anything, was seemingly the catalyst in the meetings origin. What I couldn't fathom out was if this was so, the fact that Mary's deterioration had been so severe apparently counted for nothing, even though it was reason for my reaching breaking point. To date that feeling of guilt has not left me and has since been reinforced by the pitiful inadequacy that stems from often being unable to communicate with someone you love, in the hope of perhaps directing their thoughts back to reason.

Guilty, or not, I certainly felt it. Was my eventual failure to cope surely not unexpected, in the light of the length of time I had struggled virtually alone? Comments made also quickly revealed criticism of my management of the situation, prompting me to respond that with no help whatever for in excess of three years, what chance had I? No introduction to caring is provided, you just go in at the deep end, in a sink or swim situation, and rapidly find all these leaflets that give the impression that you are supported are just so much hog wash.

Protesting this fact, I was promised by another woman that she would initiate the provision of advice on this aspect of my supposed debility to date, however, many months have now elapsed without further word and as I review my writings sixteen months later never has, or will, appear. During that course that had been held a couple of months earlier, it had apparently been very evident to one of its tutors through my body language that I was going under, but it altered nothing and it was only then and by chance that I found I apparently had a Social worker! Upon entering the room one morning, an attractive mural was found displayed on one wall which depicted the path of Alzheimer's. Upon enquiry I was told it had featured at a discussion held the previous day, but I had not been made aware of it. Much was made now too at this 'Best Decisions' meeting, that a previously mentioned organisation might have helped me.

Not much, from what you have read earlier and whilst at the meeting I cited the fact that I had responded to a recent letter stating specific times I would be available to take a call, but over seven or more weeks I had heard nothing. Oh! that person is very busy they said. She certainly must be, for several further months would elapse while I waited. There is I note never any delay, however, in sending out glossy brochures detailing various functions, where the supposed important and famous are pictured being wined and dined, or any shortage of draw ticket books and other fundraising materials. I am sorry if this is contrary to what you might expect, but I speak as I find. As for the 'Best Decisions' meeting, its outcome was that the dreaded 'Death by Separation' was now a 'fait accompli' and four weeks later its ramifications were then only all the more apparent. At the back of my mind I knew that this was ultimately the thing that was likely to happen, but now it was staring me right in the face.

All I had left as of then, was that my appeal for my wife to be transferred to somewhere nearer home was taken seriously. I appreciated that it wouldn't be easy, for the two locations nearest to home have, as I understand, to give first choice to the local hospital regarding patients discharged with nowhere to go. As Winter approached with its dark nights and poor driving conditions, let alone the travelling expense for an 80 year old on basic pension, I did not relish the prospect. The alternative was to rely on public transport, admittedly cheap through use of my bus pass, this however entailed use of four buses and over four hours of travel for each visit and some very circuitous routing through villages and narrow country lanes. Returning again to this organisation, their representative did finally come to see me and I was able to update her on both Mary's and my own situation at that time, but in the circumstances expected there was little she could offer that might be of benefit.

Forthright as ever I said so and quoted my thoughts regarding the publicity material being deceptive and its prompting false expectation. In truth one was alone and without help of any substance. Somewhat surprisingly she admitted she agreed with me, but nevertheless promised to contact me in a couple of weeks. (See the sixteen months note earlier!) A further outcome of the 'Decisions' meeting was that, in line with my wife's original respite care becoming as of that moment permanent, a smaller meeting should be held next day at her country retreat!

I was told its purpose was to tie up a few loose ends and give me the chance to find out things that were still unknown due to the emergency admission. Likewise I would get the chance to state things that I felt needed to be taken into account. Among these were that she required a visit to a dentist, also her difficulty in movement suggested that advice from a physiotherapist relating to a exercise pattern was desirable and I myself would value knowing how she was behaving during the bulk of the time, when I was not around.

This latter item was of two-fold interest to me for if I was to continue to report to her Consultant, he might well value knowing what I could tell him in comparison to the home's reporting and I could also better judge what Mary said to me as being truthful, or Alzheimer contrived to enlist my sympathy. Of course this can be arranged, it's not a problem was the ready answer, but here again several weeks elapsed without response. So was it just for the benefit of the Social Services member sitting in? As we shall see it certainly was and the list of misgivings about the care aspect in comparison to what she had promised me, quickly deepened as the weeks passed. This being so I had to remain positive, for long days, or not I did now have some time to myself, the worst of the tension had passed and there was during most visits, a period where we could continue to enjoy each other's company. I busied myself about the house on things which had been left through necessity, but in truth my heart wasn't in it without my love beside me.

JOHN ENGLAND

The Beginning of a Slow Decline

Once the first three weeks had passed, there were ominous signs that a return, albeit gradual, to former days in respect of anxiety and confusion was creeping back as each day passed. It was a disturbing thought, although not unexpected, but in the light of how wonderful those first weeks had been, any change at all brought anxiety as to where it might lead and more importantly how soon there might be a return to the traumatic situation that had existed recently at home? For myself, it was a salutary reminder too of reality for, as with any serious illness, one grasps on to the slightest hope of recovery, forgetting temporarily the cruel known outcome, in everlasting hope that the ultimate will never happen.

Indeed, the phrase 'Hope springs eternal' is so true and whatever the ailment might be, it's a case of it being hard to accept that it's happening to you rather than somebody else and there is forever hope, that at some last minute intervention might bring deliverance along the way. Science today is forever revealing greater insight into the working of our bodies and, step by step, the ravages of disease are repelled, but sadly it takes time and many must die before any cure is freely available. Meanwhile we make the best of it and do what we can to take each moment and savour it while we can.

This, however, was now and not somewhere in the future, but despite the decline there remained the chance to spend a little quality time together. During the four hours or so of my visits, which included the opportunity for us to dine together if I so wished, we could chat, watch DVDs and have tea and biscuits, even have a cuddle, however, the door of the room had to remain open and if it were closed even inadvertently, one quickly got the feeling that you had committed a crime.

Good too was the fact that the daily papers I now brought out from home were now apparently read, as were the copies of her favourite magazine in which interest had resumed, but around noon, or soon after on many days, the dreaded 'Sundown Syndrome' would return to blight the remainder of the visit by those endless questions resulting from an overwhelming anxiety that took hold of her. The day to day intensity varied, and sometimes it was subdued by painfully recounting the events relating to her lost years of memory, but, on others, it forced me to take my leave for an earlier bus home, just to enable me to recover. Once through the portals of an institutional life and back in reality, I gained a breath of fresh air and could think more of the direction of my own health and well-being. With my own medication now taken and not missed and admittedly far less stress, I had begun to pick up the pieces where the daily routine was concerned.

JOHN ENGLAND

My Cautious Building Anew

Sticking, despite the opposition to it, to a visit on every other day, there was now time to catch up on some of the household tasks for so long neglected and to begin a taming of the jungle that had once been a garden. This was fine where the daylight hours were concerned, for whilst working the mind was occupied and time flew by, but once the late afternoon's meal had been prepared, consumed and the washing up done, it was a very different story. Finding, to my mind, that other than news, there was rarely anything of substance worth watching on the television, the evening hours and eventual preparation for bed were when the terrible loneliness hit me.

I had a large collection of DVDs, CDs and taped music a'plenty, but couldn't settle to them, for they were all pungent reminders of the previous shared enjoyment. There were books too, many of which deserving of reading, or rereading, but again it wasn't easy and the bookmark rarely travelled many pages. Rather, it was a case of retiring early after making preparations for the next day's visit and deciding what might be included in a 'goody bag' of well-liked things, no longer freely available within Mary's new lifestyle. She was well-nourished at her 'country retreat' for sure, and the lack of exercise meant that those 'goodies' mustn't include too much chocolate and have plenty of fruit, but sufficient to say M&S quality and ALDI's continental specialities featured greatly.

Where the days themselves were concerned, they included a few hours for her outside those four walls and into the surrounding countryside and coast. Much as I wanted to do this it was nevertheless fraught with some amount of caution as to how she might react when we returned each time to her new home. I was also keen to incorporate a trial meal out, but unsure of what might be a suitable place to take her and had solicited suggestions to this end. However when the matter was raised again, the answer I got was I don't know, I don't live around here and like most else there, there was no feedback whatever.

In fact three or four journeys out were made and quite enjoyable in the main, but once the half-way point was made and a return commenced the atmosphere rapidly changed and driving again became difficult, due to constant anxiety led questioning. The return to the premises too were difficult, for Mary often imagined she was going home and didn't at all want to go back inside the place that lay ahead. However, thankfully, she was persuaded out of the car fairly easily when I said her dinner would be waiting, or that we could go over to the duck pond first.

Few as they were, those trips revealed too how poor Mary's mobility was and I was tempted to take some Ibrufen gel on my visits, something I could use freely when at home. However, with thoughts of the previous experience regarding the other medications, I deemed I had better not in case its odour be detected! It was destined not to be the last time that medication would feature as a concern, either as an addition, or prescribed treatment, as you will see later on in this story. The weeks though were passing as I made my way out through the countryside and harvest time arrived.

It had been mid-July when crisis point had arrived and out in the real world nature moved endlessly on and man's troubles stood as nothing. As things were all I could hope for, was that there might be a rare case of a vacancy arising in the two sites nearest to our home, but there seemed little prospect from what I had been told, yet daily I was greeted by the oft repeated call as to how much longer have I to be here? Much of Mary's regular dissatisfaction resulted from the other 'guests', who should I say were a good deal further down the road than she in their own particular version of dementia. One man with staring eyes would open the door to her room and stand silently glaring at her.

I could certainly see Mary's point, for even when I was with her it was difficult to deal with the situation. A repeated and straightforward 'go away' with a waving of one's hand had no effect, as did 'not this room', or 'you don't belong here'. Imagining he might have served his country during past days in other lands, I also tried 'Imshe!', 'Alle!' and 'Rous!', but without success. A further unwelcome visitor would be a man who shuffled about mumbling incoherently and at other times a woman would be heard shouting 'shut up, shut up' for a considerable period.

It later turned out that she was the wife of the shuffling man. Attended by an ever cheerful soul as minder, filling the role of sheep dog with its flock; we were confronted en masse by this motley band in a corridor one day after lunch. Their presence repeated somewhat more dramatically feelings experienced earlier by Mary while she attended a day centre. Far from being at all callous or uncaring in regard to their situation, her dislike of such contact was I am sure related to my knowing how upset she would become by TV and newspaper stories of animal cruelty and child abuse and being totally unable to countenance the horror of the Holocaust.

Thus I was not surprised Mary was upset, but likewise suspected it portrayed a path which Mary feared might be her own in due course. Indeed time has shown it to be a significant factor in her acceptance or not, of being taken from the home environment and normality of its life. A further factor to emerge was related to the staff looking after her, who in fact I broadly could not fault. The expression of wanting to be 'taken away from here' which accompanied my arrival, would have inference that he, or she was unkind to her, would order her about and never answered her when something was asked.

One young lad in particular was mentioned, although as I say I did not agree, but I was only there some four hours out of every forty eight, so was it all another aspect of emotional blackmail brought about by her Alzheimer's condition? I had no way of telling, but did on various occasions counter her complaint by relating the fact that she would well know from past experience as follows: We all have good days and bad, we don't always feel good and have all kinds of cares and woes, thus they affect how we do things. These people are at work and because it's a job which ends when they go home; can never equal the response of a loved one and it's a change we must get used to.

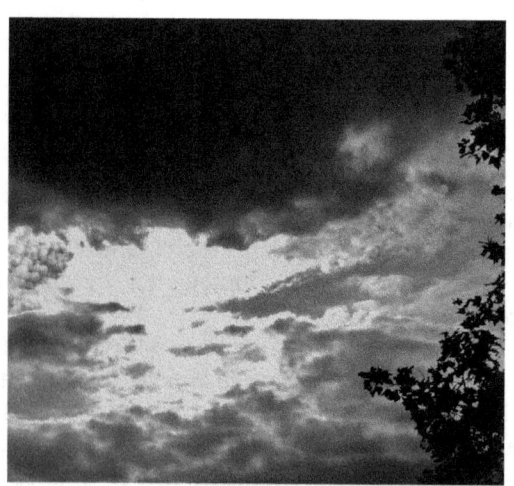

Honorable Deception?

Of course I still dare not tell Mary the truth regarding her present state, let alone the future, although I did let slip clues that might be assimilated toward any future circumstance. Instead I kept the dream alive that she might be lucky and get the chance of a move much nearer to home as she wished, but we had to be patient. Try as I may I could not bring myself to reveal that she was now incarcerated for the rest of her natural life, saying instead that this was the continuation of Respite, to allay the dread in her mind of being put away as she termed it. Time and time again this statement about this happening once before, had resurfaced at times of her condition worsening, yet the doctors had said there was nothing recorded. So were they telling the truth?

This I might never know, but I could not bear to be the one who might return her thence, concentrating instead on consolidating my love and promise never to desert her, come what may. The joy was that she now knew who I was and was desperate that we be together, rather than apart and the constant reference to her mother and happenings some 20+ years earlier were now absent, even accounting for the fact that a similar total of years memory had disappeared into thin air. Everything now related to myself being as they say 'the best thing since sliced bread' so, in comparison to the weeks of early summer, it was marvellous and at times somewhat embarrassing, for I have to admit that in general 80 year olds aren't like that.

However, we had the right to be different and I made it my business to let her know that the new existence she had, was doing Mary great good and had given a reprieve which was almost unknown with Alzheimer's.

This half a life was now better than none and it was time not to worry, she should just sit back and let it happen, rather than risk losing what had been gained so unexpectedly. For my part I both knew and understood what was best for Mary, but trying to get this absorbed by someone who forgot what has been said by the time you've taken the next breath, was next to impossible and remains so.

It was something similar where officialdom was concerned, for again having no response from the so called social worker for a couple of months, out from the blue came one from another who had supposedly now taken over, the original having been moved elsewhere (by somebody's foot I hope)! She being obviously not aware of recent events, I wrote back advising her of what had happened, asking if she was therefore still relevant and if so what she might do to assist me? Yes you've guessed it already, two further months towards Christmas passed and I was still ignored. Well not entirely, for there was a large envelope crammed with events a Carer might attend, as well as a book of draw tickets and even a sizeable collection box one could construct!

Cheeky blighters, I thought, after what I had experienced, so there's no prize for guessing where they were consigned. Where the local authority was concerned it certainly looked to be a similar case when my advising of the change of residence was concerned, however, they at least did finally respond without any correspondence. Just a sheet of bare facts without any explanation, other than it was obvious that an expected major Rate hike re my single occupancy for the current year was thankfully absent. The County Council in comparison were far more organised where supply of forms relating to costs for the care home were concerned, including return of my own original documents and those relating to Power of Attorney (now relevant).

They likewise advised details of who should be contacted where Pensions and Pension Credit were concerned and were so organised with no music while you wait and a real person to speak to, that I warmly congratulated them on that point. If you've ever dealt with them and sadly most people have; it's far different with the Work and Pensions numbers, which I duly rang and had seemingly endless music on both, before giving all the relevant information and answering any question asked. The outcome? Nothing, nix, zilch, call it what you like. Papers which I understood were to be sent never arrived and with October's days slipping by, I was dammed if I was going to go through all that paraphernalia again!

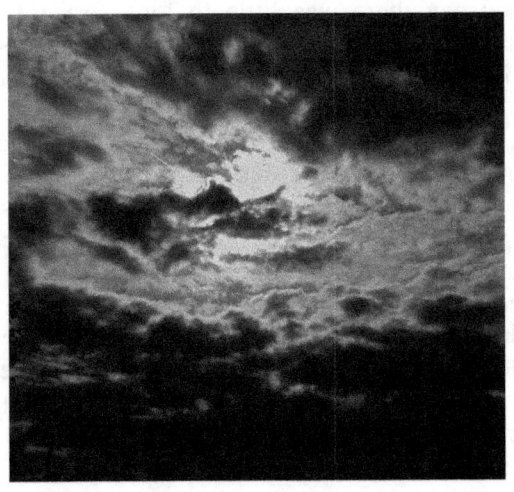

There is a God after all!

Meanwhile, the visits every second day continued and were accompanied by the niggles of vanishing laundry, never really getting questions answered and other aspects which spoilt the all over high standard of the site. I had no idea how long it might last and just kept hoping, knowing full well that the onset of Winter would surely herald increased difficulty in regard to travel. Nothing was ever done about my request for a physiotherapist visit to suggest exercises and neither was my wanting any money matter to be transparent ever realised. As day succeeded day there was little to look forward to then, completely out of the blue, the phone rang as I was preparing my evening meal and everything changed in that instant.

It was Social Services with news of a vacancy at the location I had asked for, some five minutes from home when the traffic is favourable, and served by a bus route that stopped close by! It seemed the Social Worker was more amazed than I, commenting that she had clearly imagined a year hence and still no vacancy, for normally it just didn't happen like this. I was instructed to visit the Care Home to see the accommodation and prepare to transfer my wife the next day if all was agreeable! It was indeed most agreeable and unbelievable, so could anyone really imagine I would not say yes and then quietly thank God.

In the light of anything unforeseen occurring at the last moment it must remain a secret from Mary and I was longing to see the look in her eyes when she was told the news. I courageously volunteered to go out to collect her, knowing full well a further move so relatively soon after the emergency one, was tempting fate somewhat, despite expecting her to be joyful at the outcome. If all went well the transfer could be completed within 45 minutes before she had much chance to take it all in, but that fellow Murphy arrived on the scene as one might guess, proving the view gained of the establishment was not undeserved.

We waited for laundry and expenses to be sorted out etc, but mainly for medication to be found, until I began to despair of completing the journey, for the constant delay was building Mary's tension. Eventually able to leave, only some ten minutes would elapse before we were back with 'What will mother say' etc, and I'm afraid I had to read the riot act and threaten to stop the car and leave her at the side of the road, before the torrent of confusion could be terminated somewhat to allow me to concentrate on my driving. Upon arrival the various acceptance routines were duly completed and I was told I could make only a short visit next day so as to allow her to settle in, something I was more than pleased to comply with. Now in an upstairs room of a small dementia unit as one of several others, her accommodation was with five others and had both a kitchen/diner and lounge area along, with its own laundry.

Like the original location it was local authority run and very well appointed, scrupulously clean and the quality of food would once more prove to be excellent. It only remained to see if this second move might continue the previous improvement, for everything depended upon it and only if it endured might the benefits of being so much closer to home be realised. Start as you mean to continue, I thought, so leaving her alone for one other day after that of the brief visit I recommenced my alternate day routine.

Without the hours taken up by travelling it was immediately more convenient, but even so I needed to counter any further insistence from Social Services regarding the fact that I should not visit so often. A quick calculation of the hours I had already been spending with Mary compared with those in any forty-eight, showed this only amounted to 10% and this was by no means a high proportion. Now this had undoubtedly improved, but it was only up to 12.5% and still a pitiful amount when looked at in reverse and we see that 87.5% of our married life is still spent apart.

Of course I have to admit I have gained substantially in having some time to myself, which is all very well when there are things to do that occupy the mind. However, take any evening and overnight, let alone a day confined to four walls by inclement weather and it's a rather different story, for I miss Mary terribly and cannot but rue the fact that Alzheimer's has taken away the life we had and shared so agreeably! Life isn't about what we want though is it and what we get we must be thankful for, so I'll continue now by writing more in the present tense than previously was the case and throughout it will be reinforced the overriding question at the back of the mind:

How Long will it Last?

To this day about eleven weeks later, things haven't been too bad at all considering that we are now well into the dark nights and that dreaded Sundown Syndrome thus features the more strongly. Once more dare I say against the odds, that the second move has not seriously disturbed what I have come to regard as a distinct reprieve, something that doesn't fit in to the expectation that you don't get better with Alzheimer's and the fact that the condition is terminal, although generally not spoken of as such. For now though I will leave Mary's condition for a while to catch up on some of the wider aspects of the officialdom aspect, which goes hand in hand with our change of lifestyle; for while Mary continues free of any responsibilities, these have returned to blight any easing of my previous burden.

Having notified all the relevant departments, week after week went by as if I had never told anyone. What I did know through its mention in County Council paperwork, was that as of now I'm apparently supposed to be classed as being single with a separate pension credit for each of us, so thus the question arose, do I now lose the Marriage Allowance? What I do know is that the Attendance Allowance has still not been stopped from our joint account, so well over £1,200 will have to be paid back before long.

Also because certain of my papers relating to my pension were never returned from the group that assist in these matters when urgently required by the County Council, I haven't a clue as to how much else paid into the account is mine, or will have to be paid back. This is further complicated, in that the monthly bills I pay the County Council as contribution for Mary's care, now have a sum added to cover expenses such as her hairdressing etc. As I understood it when completing the forms, this was allowed out of her pension, however, it is as I say now added so it leaves two unanswered questions. Firstly did that total as I thought now exceed her actual pension and, if so, why am I as a so called single man, apparently paying it from my basic pension?

Knowing this type of situation couldn't go on much longer I decided to again ask for help from the practice advice team and duly had a visit from one of their members whom I had met earlier on a previous occasion. It was certainly a great help, for this gentleman was most thorough and with study of all the paperwork that I could muster, soon saw things which were amiss. He was able to stop the wrongful payment of attendance allowance, finding it was not due to my notice of change being unrecorded, but an awaited notification by the care home. Likewise the local authority had noted my report, however, not apparently told their finance department. I was also to learn that it is the habit of the Pensions Department to normally allow twelve weeks to elapse, before replying!

However, it took some time before he could fathom out what exactly was wrong with the figures charged in relation to care, but something certainly was, and it required rectification. This error was amplified within the next bill and the amount increased dramatically to exceed what I knew for certain could be Mary's highest pension amount! I had agreed to continue paying whatever was asked upon the promise it would be sorted out over time, for as I have said that authority had been refreshing to deal with. As for the fact that I appeared also to be paying this allowance for her within these amounts, he imagined it related to her amount of pension credit being assumed ahead of such calculation being decided.

Thus I was advised to await the New Year to see how things settled down, when if required he would come for a further visit. Only a few days were to pass before a letter arrived from the pension credit department to say a visit would be made by one of their staff to ascertain the situation in respect of my own and my wife's entitlements. This too was most efficient in its nature, so I then looked forward to the previous chaotic situation being resolved early in the New Year. All I ask is that I get what I'm entitled to, nothing more and as someone who endeavours to keep a tidy ship where money is concerned, I don't like not knowing what I can afford to spend at any one time.

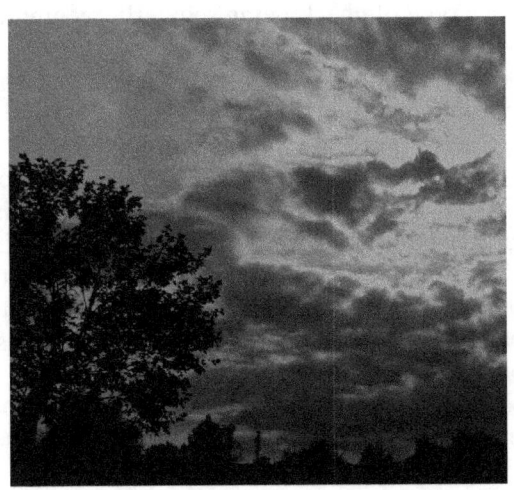

Unnecessary Aggravation

In comparison to the expected result of those two visits, I was again thoroughly disgusted by the way I was treated by my local surgery, which I detail as follows and which was relative to both my own and Mary's health. In regard to myself and despite visiting at the time of her admission to full time care and being told at that time by two doctors not to hesitate if I had problems, my own doctor was most unhelpful. When asked if he would give judgement on large warts on my shoulders, he refused, despite this type of check being regularly recommended in the press.

Secondly in respect of a leg problem which had been ongoing for around two to three years, he had no interest when I reported it intensifying of late. When pressed in regard to it being cause for concern when added to pedal control while driving, he did eventually issue me with a prescription. Having agreed to see what difference there might be, this was collected from the chemists on my way home, however, upon reading the small print accompanying it (always a wise thing to do), I was to find it was only an anti-depressant!

Needless to say I was disgusted and it will be a long time before I see him again, as for the pills, they went straight down the toilet. It was similar to another occasion years back when, in the early throws of prostate problems and water infections, another doctor upon my relating what I was experiencing as clear evidence that infection was present; brusquely dismissed my plea, saying only he alone would be the one to know when a water infection was present!

I wasn't taking that for sure and promptly told him. If he'd had one as I had, on and off over more than three years he would certainly know that I knew far better than he, what I was talking about! Needless to say I've also avoided ever seeing him again! The simple task of obtaining my regular medication each month likewise became difficult. Unable to use Mary's blue badge, and away from the house 50% of days, I provided the chemist with an alternative address for them to be delivered to, but still received notes saying you were out when we called. Fed up with this three months running I called in to see if the matter could be rectified. Imagining this to be a simple matter, especially when 'the computer' was mentioned, it took twenty minutes of consultation among the staff and the answer?

Only if you ring us each time you put a prescription in and then ring us again to advise that we have to deliver and where to, every single time! God help us what is the world coming to? Plus I had to tell them about a dozen times that the address I'd chosen would definitely have someone at home; for that person is virtually house bound! What happened to courtesy and a desire to seek any opportunity that might bring your customers regularly. As for the computers that always seem to be 'down', their operatives are wholly lost without them.

Needless to say I don't bother any longer. A stamped addressed envelope is provided and when the paperwork is returned, it's a simple matter of me going to a chemist where I can park without a problem and thus that well-advertised Pharmacy has lost my trade. As if that wasn't enough to provide hindrance, around that time I also delivered a letter to Mary's doctor to the surgery in respect of two additional prescription needs, one of which she had required before. In the letter I cited a long existing agreement signed by my wife saying I might act on her behalf, something that is now enhanced by possession of power of Attorney.

Did I get a reply of any kind? Despite politely requesting his consideration of the matters, not a word of reply was received, prompting me to think its fate had been similar to that mentioned earlier; when it was later found to have been filed away without being seen by the doctor! The answer was to advise my experience to the home and ask it to make an approach to see if they might fare better and in fact they did for a while, but the best course of action, is to steer clear of the location if at all possible.

A New Phase

Not long after Mary arrived at her new home I was pleased to receive notification of a new appointment with her psychiatrist, thus after a lengthy break during which time much had happened, continuity could be resumed. He was again most thorough, taking time to see what she could tell him of how she felt, as well as being aware of my reporting. He appeared to be well-satisfied, that even allowing for the two changes of location within a relatively short time, the improvement in her behaviour was maintained. Upon my reminding that it was now around a year since he had completed the last memory test he agreed to do another, finding only a small drop from 24 to 22, which indicated favourably.

There was more good news too, for most unexpectedly he also decided to discharge her back to her own GP, telling her that he visited the home on occasion and when there, would pop in to have a chat. It provided me with the ideal opportunity to ask if bearing this decision in mind, might there be a chance that my wish to extend taking Mary out for a ride to include a few hours at home one day as an experiment. It was then around three months since she had last been in the house and telling her about her clothes, or plants and showing her pictures didn't alone satisfy her interest.

Yes, I could take her for he had no objection, but not for another two to three months! As such that was a bit of a damper, for Mary had a birthday coming up within that period and it would also include Christmas and New Year, but I could understand his caution. A couple of weeks later this was, however, ideal conversation matter to flaunt at a follow up meeting with Social Services, who maintained an attitude similar to the 'no fraternisation' policy following the war years. I was strengthened in my resolve to give Mary the chance of a visit all the more, in the light of the home likewise reporting on how well she was adjusting to her new surroundings.

These new surroundings, although being something she had been looking forward to gaining, now though seemed of little consequence within her conversation. I certainly could not fault them in general terms, the room was comfortable, the food was excellent and it was really all I hoped it would be and, instead of the former four plus hours of travel through country lanes, it was possible to do it in five minutes, traffic permitting. Only laundry was problematical, for having clearly marked all the clothing I deemed fit to take and there only being a handful of other ladies in the unit they had a habit of regularly disappearing, or were replaced by unmarked items belonging to others, often far smaller.

Given time I was sure that would sort itself out and, if anything, I had difficulty keeping up with the large number of different faces where the staff was concerned. I always feel more confident whenever I get the chance to get to know someone, but the one or two I started to relate to would disappear for a couple of weeks before being seen again. Rightly or wrongly I've got the impression that it's this way for the benefit of the incumbents, who by seeing an ever changing number, are kept on their toes as it were and this is in line with thought that dementia sufferers often relate far better, behaviour wise, to those who are not like myself a loved one.

That seems to be proven in that the scraps of information I receive about her, are sometimes very different to what Mary tells me regarding how she feels and as I have said, I believe there are many days when I get a dose of what I have termed emotional blackmail. It's usually when I first walk in the door in the main, such as 'I don't like it here', 'they are talking about me'; but I notice that if I don't rise to the bait it often quickly dissolves, so I honestly don't think it is of any great substance. It's not that I don't believe her, but this is not her real self and reason is hard to come by when someone is in some kind of dream world for much of the time, the depth of which is totally unfathomable.

The gradual decline continues of course and the best time is the morning, however, bearing in mind we are now well within the days of the dark nights, much relates to that sundown aspect kicking in ahead of noon on many days. The most reliable gauge of how Mary is can very quickly ascertained by the number of times her mother features in the conversation, but this isn't the only source of her confusion. Many times I'm left speechless at statements that arise from nowhere, such as where did I sleep last night, is there a toilet here, or where do I go for my food then?

God only knows I've lost count of how many times I've gone through where she is, why she's there, etc, and how long it is since her mother departed this world. I try my hardest to get her to sit back and 'let it happen' rather than keep worrying, but it's an uphill and never-ending struggle. With Mary having virtually no memory, my story is and will remain, that she was so ill that it was affecting her physical health (heart) and had to be brought to a special unit dealing with dementia (not an old peoples home, not a hospital etc), and this is taken without question. What is really important is that she now knows who I am and wants me by her side, something that still gives me the chance to lavish the love and care that she needs to assuage the horror that lurks in her mind from long past days.

For my part probably the most difficult thing is dealing with the sudden mood swings that arise without warning and which relate almost exclusively from anxiety and are no doubt accelerated by the loss of any readily accessed memory. One will often be able to listening to music, or be watching a DVD, enjoying the fact that the experience is shared as in past times, but as of say the flick of a switch all is lost by 'I'll have to be getting back!', or something similar. As such it is the precursor of a lengthy insistence that we are back in her other world of the 1980s, with her mother alive, a motorised cycle and a house to look after and no amount of persuasion to the contrary is achieved, unless one can break the spell by some means; but how!

If you are lucky someone might come in and break the spell, to ask would a cup of tea be welcome, or to return some washing; but other than that it's a long uphill task to regain some normality. The best policy is to endeavour to keep calm, when actually you are gutted that what was going so well is now down the drain and begin for the umpteenth time to remind her that in reality all is well. It will solve the problem sometimes, but more often than not even though you think you are getting somewhere, a breath is taken and we are back to square one in continuing belief that we are in her world of somewhere in the 1980s, before we even met, or even earlier!

One Small Step, One Giant Leap?

This being so, perhaps the hardest thing to combat is the fear that grips Mary as to her being in danger of some kind or another, especially of darkness and being left alone when it's time for me to leave her. All of these of course would come to a head the more so when the chance to visit her real home came and if this was to be associated with her forthcoming birthday, there was need to seek the opinion of the manager of the home before it was attempted. After so much negativity on the part of others, it was indeed a revelation to find that she was very supportive of my wishes. The chance had to be taken, if it failed at least it would have been tried, but my real surprise was that ahead of my saying anything about perhaps making it a weekly event if it were successful; she envisaged visiting twice a week as a possibility rather than once!

This was fine if it worked it would be wonderful and should it be so; why on earth hadn't I had the courage to ask earlier! Thus somewhat sustained, I was never the less anxious, for although the first visit would be on her birthday and chance of success aided perhaps by the presence of others; what might happen when it was time to return her to her new abode. When that day dawned I was encouraged in that it was a rare bright day, so with luck the 'sundown' aspect might be minimised, although when I arrived to collect Mary she seemed surprised to see me and had obviously forgotten where she was going. (A complete reversal of many days when shoes are on and coat ready when no trip is envisaged!)

That being so, there was too one very good sign, in the fact that once in the car she said she realised her mother must be dead, for in being over twenty when she was born, she would be at least 106 now! Interestingly this was not an isolated case of being very capable of reasoned thinking, for there had been other recent examples. When I had said one afternoon about her being half way to 90 (meaning that 85 would be half way to 90, while in her current 80s), she quickly responded - 'but I'm much older than 45'. Perhaps the best one was when I was recently taking her along the corridor for some exercise. From nowhere an unknown lady Carer arrived asking somewhat sharply where were we going?

Before I had any real chance to explain that this movement was authorised, Mary responded with great vigour as follows - 'It's all right, when we get to Africa we'll ring you!' There have been others too like while we were out for a ride in the country and a field with a fair quantity of geese prompted me to pause, for they are not a normal sighting hereabout, my contemplation of the unusual aspect only, was accompanied by 'They'll be fattening them up for Christmas' and this from someone who has no concept of time any longer until she is prompted.

The birthday visit to our home having been judged fairly successful, Christmas was not too far ahead, however, any hope that on both days someone else would be there and thus minimise the chance of Alzheimer's spoiling it; went rapidly down the drain when an urgent hospitalisation of the intended cook for that day took place. This gave rise to thought that rather than the rigmarole of taking her back and forth during the two days, might there be less disruption if she were to come home and stay overnight? In all it didn't go too bad, although it wasn't perfect, but successful enough to prompt thought of a similar arrangement for New Year's Eve and the day itself.

This in fact was confirmed when day one could only be described as heaven, for it brought memory of how things used to be and how precious that time had been, when Alzheimer's was only something you read of in the papers. The second day, however, would bring difficulty, especially in the latter part of the afternoon when return was due to the full time care location. Quite naturally Mary did not want to go back and the dark winter days did nothing to help in this situation. Around this time, the two days of the week when I visited the home, now went fairly well and many a hour was spent together listening to music and watching all kinds of DVD.

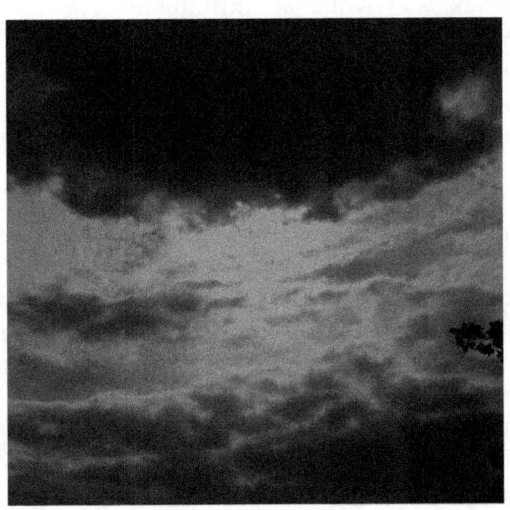

Spring to Summer - 2011

Here though there was further reminder and an important one too; that one shouldn't be complacent for with somewhat frightening swiftness, the situation could still change rapidly. In an instant one was back to suffering the relentless onslaught of a being who has lost their real identity of today and is locked in a world they knew more than twenty years previous. Any attempt to bring Mary back to reality was usually entirely fruitless, for sublimely confident of what she was saying, she would fiercely argue black was white ad infinitum.

Whatever, but the fact was that the joy of those precious moments when normality had returned, would be more than compensation for the remainder, so regardless of what might be the outcome, I decided to make the weekend visit to home fairly a regular event. In this I shared the view of the manager that she really did deserve it and it might help allay her growing number of references to being put away, something as I have said which must never be confirmed. Mary was certainly at times very confused and the memory was chaotic to say the least, but she wasn't stupid by any means and as the weeks passed she certainly sized up her surroundings and those immediately within it faithfully.

The other five from what I could see were best described as waiting to die, for they would sit for hours to stare blindly ahead, or if placed in front of a television would fill what mind they had with what went on in front of them without response; let alone ever be seen to read a book, or paper as far as I could see. There was certainly no *Rising Damp, Steptoe, Hello Hello,* or *Faulty Towers* that Mary could lose herself in, no Pavarotti, Orchestral highlight, or landscape of distant shores, in what remained of their lives! Their only alternative to the television was the seemingly unending repetition of 1940s songs retailed by the likes of Max Bygraves. Obviously well-intentioned, rather than promote any mental stimulation they, to my mind, only hastened the decline of those unfortunately in earshot.

Indeed Mary now often wanted to know why she was there at all for, in comparison to them, she felt all right except that she was deluded memory wise in thinking she still kept house, went into town and still went shopping etc, due to the Lewy bodies presence in her brain, which still has no answer. To all questions regarding why she is there residing in her 'flat' and not at home, I cite the doctor's reasoning that it will most importantly maintain the status quo. He is seeking to maintain her present condition for as long as possible and that it is neither an old peoples' home, or a hospital.

I repeatedly remind Mary that it is a small County Council unit catering for those like herself, who have Alzheimer's in one form of another. She should be thankful that its routines have allowed her to gain significant improvement from that of last year, when physical harm through the return of former heart problems and falls, was the cause of great concern to both of us. As I now write this, some seven or eight weekends have been spent with Mary and I at home, but once more I'm afraid that after an idyllic Saturday from mid-morning onward, Sunday was difficult to deal with and I am constantly anxious as to how long it might continue.

Not only did I get mother, step father, the house, the bike and this fictitious step mother she most certainly never had, but I was back reliving those bad days of last year, when I'd have given anything to get out of the room just for a few precious seconds. Could it be I wondered, that perhaps Social Services were right after all, when insisting that I should minimise my visits, for with Mary's surroundings changing regularly, it could be counter-productive in unsettling her. I bravely put this to her, but the response was that she had enjoyed herself and didn't think she had done any wrong; it was I alone that had spoilt things!

Returning to what I said earlier in relation to the chance ending of mood swings by someone entering the room, the opposite too, was in fact what happened on more than one occasion during recent weeks. It was all going so well, but the DVD was lost and the music forgotten, upon entry of a Carer to administer medicines and another later to see what she would like for lunch. It is really like treading on eggshells and whatever you do you can't win and seemingly never will, for you are shadow boxing an unknown which you can never get the measure of and this gives rise to an immense feeling of helplessness.

However, leaving the one to one encounters for a moment, I will return briefly to the ongoing saga with officialdom. The twists and turns of this monster continued into the early months of this year. Despite having a home visit from both a representative of the Local Authority and from Pensions Credit, with all the relevant paper work on show each time, the Local Authority firstly had myself recorded as the one with a disability and I was secondly listed as still getting a Carer's Allowance. Thanks to a great deal of help from a gent from the County Council Practice Advice Team, much though has been rectified and at long last the financial situation has been eased with the payment of various moneys owed to me. It's a sign of how chaotic things are that this gent who as I say has visited twice, still said if it still wasn't right at the end of the financial year, I must call him for further assistance.

JOHN ENGLAND

The Big Squeeze

This, however, was happily not required, yet great as his contribution is to many like myself who find themselves somewhat overwhelmed by the plethora of official forms and their complexity, he advised that where Governmental decisions regarding expenditure were concerned, he was expected to be one of the first casualties in the round of spending cuts! Ah! yes spending cuts!

Their being necessary, or not, it's the speed and ruthlessness of the decisions that make one blanche and while speed cameras, libraries and school crossing ladies grab the headlines, our particular County Council is one of those which plans to dispose of its entire Care Home holding by closure, or transfer into the private sector as a matter of priority, irrespective of the fact that number requiring care are increasing and place availability is diminishing. Their statement that nothing would be done without full consultation cut little ice though, at an initial meeting set up for friends and family, to meet with around half a dozen officials. It was certainly a foregone conclusion that very soon each of us and particularly our loved ones would have to endure likely upheaval to the well run and caring homes, on the grounds that facts and figures for expected expenditure to maintain statutory regulations were prohibitive.

Given this, what hope was there that they might be taken over by the private sector and whatever the result was, both patient and family would therefore presumably suffer upheaval and loss of a most satisfactory existence.

Much of the meeting time was lost by the concentration upon illustration of new build private care homes and the presence of one man, whose persistent arguing with the individual representatives of the Council, thereby greatly curtailed the time allowed for questions. It was very clear that questions needed answers and my particularly input was should not Care Homes take preference over Council services not traditionally supplied.

One prominent example was one where a Council service was in open competition with long term private companies of varied and considerable expertise. As such it was more than conspicuous by the style and manufacturer of its vehicles, leading to expectation that its growth was down to a severe bout of Empire Building on the part of the department head concerned. In short we are talking in terms of children being taken to school in vehicles which are more fitted for use as away games transport, by nationally known top football clubs!

Again I have digressed from my main theme, but so much cutting has been made without due thought to its value in the community as a whole and as a sample I'll cite pensioners restricted to travel after 0930. It doesn't help workers one little bit who usually go by car, but hinders mothers with young children who travel by bus, leaving one lightly used bus being followed twenty minutes later by one that's packed, as they say 'to the gunnels'. As the weeks have gone by for the families and the care workers themselves who stand the risk of loss of their jobs, almost no mention of what is planned has been noted in the press.

What has received good publicity, engendered campaigns and fulsome radio and TV coverage, is library closure, cuts to school crossing persons and similar more run of the mill subjects, which because they currently affect far more people, are likely to survive the upheaval brought about by the Budget Deficit Country wide. Where self-preservation is king, and sadly it is as an outcome of our present day life style; the Care Home subject like dementia itself, is something to be swept under the carpet as it were, as someone else's problem. Indeed cancer had the same treatment for years, bringing back thoughts of long past days, when unfortunates variously afflicted, rang a bell and shouted 'unclean' as they went their way.

Ask most people what they know about dementia and they'll probably say they know of someone who had it, but are dead now! That's certainly not the case for the six to eight hundred thousand that have it today, let alone their families. From what we read, in very few years that number will double and Government will be forced to take notice! 'Not in my backyard' my foot, they are all getting old and one day not too distant it will be their turn, or that of someone dear to them and it will be a bit late to dismiss it as someone else's problem. In mid-April I received an invitation to attend a meeting at another County Council run home, although it contained no detail of what is proposed to engender a last minute change of heart on the part of the Council.

As for how I presently feel, I believe there are many well run Care Homes and private enterprise is after all part and parcel to our way of life, but instinctively I know that profit should not be a consideration where flesh and blood is concerned. I also know that Councils abide by the rules and thereby correctness is ensured to their activities throughout; whether it be standards of health, welfare, or any other aspect of the provision of a service and their workers are not only paid commensurate rates, but continually have to abide by certain rules and standards.

The public sector though sometimes maligned, is broadly accepted as a fair employer and provider of the tools for the job, something brought home to me somewhat surprisingly during an earlier employment. It was certainly a revelation, for my being privy to the thoughts of, shall I say, numerous persons of stature and rank, their conversations between themselves, without exception favoured a return to the days of Nationalisation, for the provision of mainstream needs of the populous, believing that any service relating to the needs of the wider community should be from a Nationally run organization.

Yes I do indeed mean Telephone, Post, Water, Power, Rail and Road Haulage, Health and Education. Also, I certainly don't understand why the County Councils have to fund the shortfall between care costs and what you are judged to afford. As one who was in at the beginning of the National Health Scheme in post war days, the stated concept was 'From the Cradle to the Grave', so where did that concept get lost? It's not hard to contemplate that it has much to do with the original 'Free at the point of need' now being provided to every Tom, Dick and Margaret from heaven knows where, who have never paid in over long years like we have and so it's become a kind of World Health Organisation, rather than the National Health Service it once was.

Descent into the Unknown

I've already indicated how unpredictable Mary is at present and in comparison to the recent past where there was some rather remarkable and totally unexpected improvement, I think volatile is its best current description. In truth I am forced to admit that the past two months have brought a deterioration and this is confirmed in a simple mark-up of the calendar. I introduced it last year with a simple tick for a good day and a cross for a bad and struck through the tick slightly if it was one which had become neither. During March through to July during 2010 the number of crosses gradually outnumbered the ticks until none at all remained and sadly this pattern is now being repeated during 2011.

It has meant that not only have I had to cease the few overnight weekend visits to home, but virtually cancelled bringing her home at all even for only a few hours. Although Mary says she wants to come and says she enjoys it, I'm not at all sure if she really understands, for she continually says things that indicate the loss of facts and suggest she dwells in some make believe existence for considerable periods. It's the degree of uncertainty that pervades most conversations that l find baffling, and yet as I have said she nevertheless, often remains capable of highly original thought and riposte to circumstance and remains a very good judge of character.

I now have to take it even more as one day at a time, ever hopeful, yet knowing that the more you hope the chances are that it will be disappointment that you suffer rather than joy. I've almost given up on the playing of

DVDs, for whether it's on a rare visit home, or on my visits to see her one is lucky to just get five minutes into it, when this anxiety thing cuts in and continues for the rest of the time with her. That previously mentioned Saturday was so difficult that it cancelled any chance of having Mary home on that Sunday as was intended and it left me so drained that I didn't even visit her until a couple of days had elapsed.

I spent that day instead in the garden, but I couldn't enjoy it, for I felt I had let her down and I couldn't help thinking of her perhaps somewhat recovered and sitting for long hours, wondering where I was and why I was not with her. The root of the problem is this terrible anxiety about anything and everything, which interrupts whatever interest I try to provide for her, be it film, music, photos, or conversation. The need to get back to mother or her flat, of course, predominates, also her mother not knowing that she is 'seeing me'.

Over several days, it was Mary's continuing fear that her husband would arrive and catch us together that lasted the day long and at other times she is convinced she goes to work, has been into town shopping and she knows the various the lady Carers well, having formerly worked with them at Marks & Spencers, or the Co-op! Memory it seems is comprehensively non-existent from around the mid-1980s and its current duration is at best a couple of minutes at its best. Only on very rare occasions currently is there any chance of a meaningful conversation, and there are times when anything is talked about one gets the feeling that it either isn't fully understood, or there is no interest remaining other than where she is and what she is doing there.

In fact Mary has been in that room now for almost a year, but still often asks where the toilet is (less than ten feet away), where she will spend the night and regularly imagines she has come to see me, rather than it is I that is visiting her. The loss of memory one could deal with if there was chance that a reminder of the facts would end the uncertainty, however without any instant recall, what I say is lost in the instant that the breath leaves my mouth, so what hope is there of any real and meaningful conversation, or understanding as in past times?

If one of us had been struck dumb or could no longer hear, one could manage I'm sure, but with absolutely no comprehension of what is going on in her mind other than that confusion more often than not reigns in abundance, one is again left feeling utterly useless and you wonder how much longer you can stand it. I love Mary so much and knowing the value of the wife and person she has been, one is overcome with grief that she should degenerate to this. At times you feel great tenderness, as if she is a new born infant brought forth into the world that has to be cradled in your arms, to be reassured and protected.

At others it's as if you are dealing with someone with whom you simply cannot meaningfully communicate, because neither knows a single word of the others language. You too are a victim of conscience, for when the situation deteriorates to walk away would only cause her pain, for whoever she really thinks I am, Mary continues to be desperate that I should stay. However, the longer you stay the greater the feeling of impotence and there is desperation to be away out in the fresh air and clear of the sheer mind-numbing atmosphere of it all. Not only that, but such inability to cope brings frustration, yet enduring an awful guilt if one ever gives up the struggle against this 'being' that manifests itself, where previously there was understanding, gentility and love.

Whatever, there is one overriding consideration and this is, that however jaded you have become from what I have described earlier as these relentless mind games, one must endeavour to part with tenderness and manifold expression of love, for at our age it may be the last time we are together in this world. As sure as the sun sinks and night follows day, this day will come and I could not bear us to part other than in unity, lest she be left feeling unloved and abandoned, in the purgatory in which she is perhaps immersed for many years yet.

True, Mary has put on weight due to the lack of mobility and good food inclusive of extra helpings, to such an extent that I've had to cut down the little box of goodies on each visit and boost it instead with more fruit. Apart though from her aches and pains and an increasing lack of energy, which is not that unusual for her age, Mary certainly and thankfully remains fit and without the earlier need for regular hospital visits, to various consultants as in previous years. Thus it is very likely that, although I am more than five years younger, she is quite likely to outlive me and her stay 'in captivity', if one dare put it that way, could yet be lengthy.

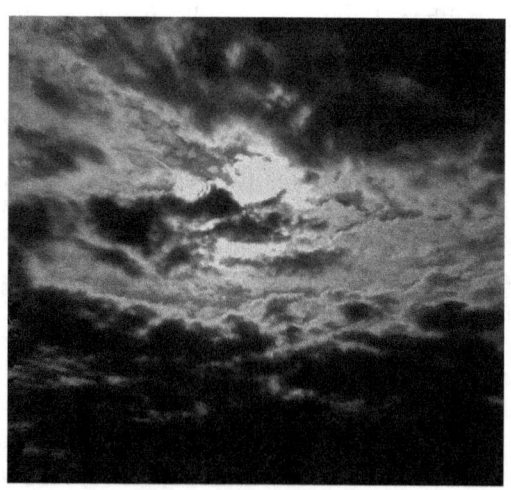

JOHN ENGLAND

In a Trice –
Sheer Joy and Complete Devastation

A few days of an earlier month as if I needed any reminder; encapsulated the agony of Alzheimer's, for it brought a glimpse of a life that once was and is now lost, to be followed immediately with the ramblings of a tortured mind wracked with anxiety and in total confusion. Easter day this year happened to fall on my birthday and there was hope that a visit home would perhaps be blessed, with a few hours as near as possible to what they used to be. Indeed they were and it was wonderful for almost six and a half hours passed during which a meal was shared, there was laughter, togetherness and hardly a word to denote the chasm that often exists. True when it was time to return Mary 'home' it wasn't quite so perfect, but it had been so good a time together, that I felt totally renewed.

Next day she was due to visit the seaside and a coach was booked for around twenty or so who were to complete the visit. I was to find it included myself, however, at mention of a sing song en route, I chickened out as they say; preferring to travel independently. It proved to be a wise decision, for arriving ahead of the group and she not remembering that I was going, it was a revelation to see the joy in Mary's face as I waited. Any reservation that I had had about getting involved therefore quickly melted and for a few hours it was even better than the previous day, for she remained happy, even excited and some mischievous humour on her part ensured laughter throughout the stay.

To say it was a tonic was an understatement, for truly I could not remember when she had been so relaxed. The welcoming cup of tea was followed by traditional fish and chips, before departing along the sea front with her in a wheelchair ahead of the others, with the idea of locating an ice cream kiosk. Quite quiet when found, we decided to pause to chat with the proprietor, my suggesting this might stimulate custom for him and indeed this was the case. Fortified with the largest '99' he could provide, it was indeed a revelation to find Mary joined in lengthy conversation to the extent that I imagined he must be thinking any ailment she had must be bodily rather than mental.

Returning to join the others, I enjoyed talking for a while to a gentleman who turned out to be like myself a family member, but Mary wanted to go back inside the building and that did I know it was to prove my undoing! I won't get caught like that twice for certain, but not used to such 'company' shall we say; I sat on a cushioned chair and in no time at all felt distinctly uncomfortable, for its previous occupant had emptied their bladder earlier whilst seated! A somewhat distasteful event obviously, but that day and the previous will remain forever with me, as full of truly wonderful and precious moments, when we shared the happiness of past days.

It would have been foolish to imagine it would last, but like the drowning man you clutch on even at straws in everlasting hope and savour every last drop of nectar that such occasions bring. I had hardly entered the room at my next visit to Mary when I sensed this day would be much different, for the uncharacteristic attitude of confusion laced with aggression was evident from the start. The DVD of *Upstairs Downstairs,* which she would normally have become engrossed in, had hardly started, before getting back to her flat, mother and all those so oft repeated demands flooded out and ruined the day. It was impossible to change the subject, there might be the odd moment when you thought there was a chance of her regaining composure, but no it got worse and worse.

Lunch time came and went and any attempt to commence the daily exercise and short walk that followed had to be abandoned in the face of an unremitting torrent of demands that she be taken home to flat, mother et al. After some four and a half hours of this, all I wanted to do was go, for it was pointless staying, but any mention of this brought remonstration as to my abandoning her, her being afraid to be alone in a strange place etc. In desperation I called in a lady Carer, who likewise tried through pleading for Mary to relax, settle down and listen to what was being said, for she had no reason to be worried. It was my cue to depart, there was a kiss and a hug and I left a couple of hours prematurely, feeling as sick as a parrot that it had come to this.

Overwhelmed by Pity

  Reaching the end of the corridor I looked back. Mary had come to the door with a look that was to haunt me throughout the whole weekend. I had deserted her in her hour of need, for whatever confusion reigned within her brain she needed me, reached out for me, as the one person remaining in the void that has developed when twenty odd years of memory dissolved virtually overnight. I blew her several kisses, but now with a door between us, like it or not I had to keep going; there was no way I could go back for it would only have prolonged the agony. Realistically with no memory once I was out of sight she would almost certainly forget I had visited.
  At least that's what I hoped, for if so that's where she has the advantage on me poor soul, for I on the other hand could only remember that parting and the shock of it, when it had been sheer heaven only relatively few hours before. Therein is the difficulty, for a statement like 'I just can't get my head round it' is so easily said, but the facts are that that you can't, for such a profound difference exists in one that you know and love, that it's almost like they have already partially died; for really they retain only a small proportion of our world. Every so often and a further weekend was such an example, the person you have known returns as they would in a dream and you enjoy that experience immensely, but it is transient and departs without warning to leave one in purgatory, caught between the heaven of the former life and the hell of their loss by a death that is yet to come.

That is how I felt for the next couple of days, wanting to hold Mary in my arms, yet almost dreading going back in fear that she remained as I had left her. Go back I did for nothing can stop me and a little later than normally, out of necessity of some shopping to find her out in the corridor being comforted by a Carer. She apparently feared I would not come and wanted desperately to get out to look for me. That being the case one would think that once there by her side she would be reassured and settle down to enjoy what we could of the day, but sadly it doesn't work like that. As days go it wasn't that bad, but throughout the memory loss and confusion together combined to produce an endless dialogue relating to why she was there, where it was, when would she be leaving, were we married, where did I live, had I seen her mother, step mother etc.

Where would she sleep tonight, why couldn't I take her with me, she would be alone, ad infinitum (or should that be ad nauseam?). It was now mid-June and I was constantly reminded of the fact that a whole year had passed since those desperate weeks of twelve months ago, when confined to what one could call a pressure cooker for so long, I was almost out of my mind. It will soon be three years since the dramatic escalation of the Alzheimer's condition and one is forced to ask one's self how much longer will it last? It's a selfish thought I know, but my life has in so many ways stopped and at this time of life, am I likely to live long enough to see it recommence?

Confined in this deadly routine I am starved of contact with the wider world and long for contact and conversation with those who minds are free from torment. A few hours with such would truly be a breath of fresh air and lift my spirits, but want as I may I cannot, for I am bound by conscience and a love so deep, that I will not leave her side for more than a few hours; however difficult it is and totally fruitless more often than not. Of late, confusion has been Mary's greatest problem, leading to the weekends at home being curtailed somewhat. It would be perhaps better described as attendance deficiency, for it is noticeably more difficult for music, or a story to be uninterrupted.

There are odd happenings too to relate, like becoming upset while briefly meeting someone she had known for many years. Breaking off the encounter as quickly as I could, I could not fathom out why this should be and was totally at a loss, to find it was due to her believing it to be the mother of her first husband! Another overnight visit produced a further instance of talking, snorting and laughing in her sleep, while limbs were active and eyes mostly open. It went on for over an hour, during which all manner of attempts were made in vain to waken her, inclusive of in desperation, holding the ringing alarm clock beside her ear! During the day that followed, I was told twice that other persons were in the room with us, something not mentioned now for several months, but yet another sign perhaps of further deterioration.

JOHN ENGLAND

The Prospects Diminish

The calendar says it's now mid-July, but in reality it's just a seemingly unending round of visits which are more unsuccessful by the day. It is tiring, dispiriting, debilitating and above all depressing, as what remains of the one that means so much to me, slips slowly and relentlessly away, to be replaced by a tortured soul. Our encounters are becoming more like a maze of contrasts to be negotiated, for Mary is desperate to be with me and utterly saddened at my departure and yet while I am with her conflicting demands disrupt conversation and all else, as she concocts all manner of suppositions devoid of any relation to reality. Such behaviour led to chaos on three recent weekends that were meant to provide her with a breath of life as it used to be. Each commenced with a ride out into the countryside, but at the first sign of my heading back towards town, her expectation was to return from where she had originally come from rather than home.

My knowing this was contrary to what had been stated only a half hour before, I pressed on hoping that upon seeing her former home she would settle, but it was not to be. Entering the house reluctantly she would not stay and insisted she should be returned, but after only 50 yards and in the middle of a difficult junction, insisted that I turn back! No way, I thought, so I continued to the care home, where she would not get out, proclaiming she would now like to go home for the intended visit. A glutton for punishment you might say, I hadn't the heart to refuse her plea to visit the following week, however, there was a similar change of mind that time and then on a further weekend we got no further than our driveway, for Mary refused to even get out of the car. The result? We returned to the Care Home and, protest or not, she went back in, although I then of course had great difficulty for as ever Mary didn't want me to leave her.

As of now she keeps asking to return home at the weekend, but once there for a few hours she will not leave and it develops into a trial of wills. The most recent of these was on a Saturday which was perfection for the first three hours and the opposite for the next four, for once she has this mood swing there's no stopping it. Visiting her on Sunday evening for two hours was again fine, but once I prepared to leave the mood turned to a mixture of sorrow and aggression, where whatever one said was turned to an accusation of rejection and betrayal.

Thirty six hours later was a repetition that led me to depart unable to withstand the relentless onslaught of twisted outpourings, which alternated between declarations of love and condemnation. I knew it would be difficult the moment I entered the room, for Mary was slumped in her chair seeming more unconscious than asleep and once more nothing it seemed could rouse her. I asked the work experience girl with her to get one of the Carers for as the minutes passed I began to wonder if this was anyway normal, for there was some loud and distorted laughter and slurred attempt at speech, as in one of the earlier night times at home. Eventually she was roused apparently none the worse for what I had witnessed, but I was concerned as to why these events took place. On mentioning my interest to a senior Carer who came to administer medication there was but a brief and dismissive reply. When people get old it's not unusual for them to often drop off into a deep sleep, so I was left none the wiser.

This then is the composition of happenings at this time, although there remain times when I can enjoy two to three hours of a visit. In general terms this is usually after

I arrive and often conversation can be so normal that I intentionally widen it to see just how varied it can be. Perhaps it's about something in the news, or maybe work I've been doing at home, but whatever it is the comparison with later behaviour is astounding. Where this is concerned and as you will have already gathered, confusion regarding her 'Mother' has recently returned with a vengeance, after a break of several months during which it did not feature. Also, despite memory being almost non-existent, one can likewise be surprised, for when a Dave Allen DVD was inserted alongside music one day last week, I was not only reminded that she had seen the sketch before, but a piece of music too!

Notwithstanding this, there are however questions as to who it is that she is with in photographs on the wall, she will ask about my wife, or indeed how my husband is! Statements that defy comprehension sometimes astound me, for they refer to things which have never related to our lives. Recent examples of this have been talk about her needing to get the boys ready for football and arrange for money to be paid to a university. Notwithstanding this and another amusing one about a picture of an elephant that was supposedly on the wall, but one specific factor causes us both a great difficulty of late.

This relates to the fact that we now lead separate lives and what was originally accepted as far as this is concerned, is now replaced with a vivid realisation that she will remain like this until she dies. During the past year there has seemingly been a quiet acceptance of her new lifestyle and throughout if the subject has arisen, I have said clearly that there is no cure and we must sadly accept that baring miracles, I cannot say other than that. Mary is, however, patently very different to the other five women residents in her wing and therein is perhaps the nub of the problem; I can but guess.

As I have said before they are seen to be passive, either sat at table for endless hours gazing into space, or likewise in front of the television, apparently saying virtually nothing unless prompted by a Carer. To me it's as if their particular malady has shut them down, are no longer capable of expressing themselves and without initiative, they wait for direction and submit without question. This is a world away from Mary's situation and given that she can be so totally confused, has lost so much of her memory and suffers great anxiety; she does retain spirit and determination.

This active rather than passive aspect is even expressed at the times of confusion, for not only does Mary often believe that she keeps house, goes shopping, works even and remains capable of organising things, but more importantly wants to! Mary isn't in pain so she doesn't feel ill, remains actively aware of things like cleanliness, tidiness, looking her best regarding clothes, hair and make-up. She also enjoys her food, can feed herself and remains acutely aware of inconsistencies in others, regarding their work and behaviour.

Treading Water

    Thus muddled, as Mary often is, the overriding influence currently is as follows. She cares greatly about where she is, why she is there, when it will end, what she did to make it happen and above all is certainly aware of what has been lost by her present predicament. In short the others express submission to the inevitable, either voluntary, or through the progression of their particular illness and thus appear already dead. My Mary on the other hand, could be said to fit the phrase, dead but won't lie down and I'm sure it is very much a result of her experiences before we met! As I have said, she would never speak of them, and still won't, despite my repeated asking, but the doctors won't say and whatever they were, it's clear her life was transformed by our meeting.

    Despite Mary not remembering the details, it's ingrained in her mind that our years together brought heaven in place of hell. The thought that it is now lost terrifies her, for obviously it was of comparatively short duration (around 17 years) and what she valued so much is now gone. I alone know how it hurts, for such feelings are only shared when we are alone together and it is painful to experience the sadness that grips her while trying to understand what she might have done to snatch it from her grasp, just as life was at last worth living. She cannot bear for me to leave her and clings to the very last second at our parting endlessly asking one more time when I will return. No matter how difficult the previous hours may have been, the idea of parting crystallises her thoughts and it is so painful to her that tears accompany pleas to remain just that little bit longer.

What pitiful few there are in the outside world who ask of Mary, are no doubt well-meaning in their suggestions of what I should do at this time, but they are not involved and their ideas lack feeling. I am told I should only visit rarely, not take her out and certainly not bring her home and if I do visit should leave suddenly, because she will quickly forget that I've been. Sadly their tidy solutions remind very much of the biblical tale relating to those that passed by on the other side and heaven help those that might depend on them at some future time. Mary may well be overcome by her illness for long periods, but at others retains remarkable clarity as to her true feelings and often expresses great charity and foresight.

Despite my being with her remaining the linchpin of her existence as it were, Mary will often say that I should leave her, for I would be better to find someone else, rather than waste my time remaining with her. Likewise she continually links this with the subject of money, saying I should take it and enjoy myself while I can. When I protest that this will not happen under any circumstances and that she has made charitable decision within her Will in regard to the latter, she is adamant it should be done. Of course nothing will change and my vow to love and cherish in sickness and in health, till death us do part is pre-eminent and will certainly stand the test of time.

I don't care, confusion or not I can tell sincerity and there remains within my Mary a high proportion of down-right common sense, which is revealed during her periods of lucid personal conversation. Thus I will not exit suddenly, certainly not leave her for days on end, or do anything else that might distress her further. There is also another aspect to consider, for not being passive as are others, Mary realises she is constrained, restricted, incarcerated, even imprisoned. Forgetting her lack of mobility and sensory deprivation, she wants to go out by herself, wishes to go with me to events as we used to and even wants us to go away on holiday!

When told it cannot be Mary asks why not, for she hasn't done anything wrong, so why should she be imprisoned! She certainly feels as if she is and often asks if she will die there. A difficult one that, for in fact she is certainly likely to and will either die there, or in hospital. Having read these last few paragraphs you will perhaps understand a few of the ramifications of what I have termed my fight with Alzheimer's. Has what I have said not proved it wrong to conclude that such cases can be quietly put away, while you get on with life. Some perhaps depending on the nature of their debility, but certainly not Mary, who alone out of the other five can share meaningful conversation with her Carers as I have said.

Mary clings to me as sole remnant of those comparatively few years during which she enjoyed a life without anger, arrogance and poverty of feelings. In their place there was freedom, happiness, security and love, so whilst she is presently restricted and without hope, no wonder every moment we are together is precious; even if I also act as receptacle for her frustration with confusion. Something else too gives me much thought and it relates to the varying pattern of Mary's behaviour, seeing that it is widely recognised that you don't get better once you have Alzheimer's. As you will have read there have been significant changes along the way, those immediately following her being taken from home being the most significant. Also I have said that despite the increasing number of years now passed since it was diagnosed; the deterioration I speak of is in many ways a change of emphasis, or partial reversion to former aspects. Likewise these times that I have mentioned during which we talk quietly and she is extremely lucid, are far more prevalent than say six months ago. Twelve months ago of course they were impossible, so one is completely lost when trying to comprehend the disease's progress, let alone what lies ahead in future months.

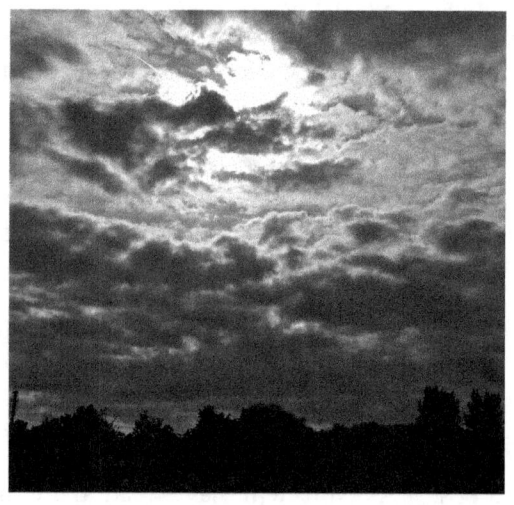

JOHN ENGLAND

Two Lives on Hold

My own existence fairs similarly where the outside world is concerned, as I adjust as best I can to what has been and remains a long drawn pattern of bereavement. There are long hours in an empty house, Winter is approaching and darkness arrives at an alarming rate. There's no fun in dining alone day after day and at every turn I'm reminded of what we have lost and how short a time we were together here. There has of course been time to get a few jobs done and the garden is where I've spent the highest number of hours, but my increasing years mean that by lunch time tiredness overtakes me and four walls again become my prison. As you might guess, the woman from that already mentioned organisation never did return, but although I shouldn't appear on their records any longer the local authorities Carers organisation still sends its literature.

Most recently this comprised a long list of events and activities that Carers could engage in and in particular details of a pamper session, though what males might want with eyebrow shaping, yoga, Indian head massage, meditation, or hot stone therapy; entirely escapes me! The intended change, namely divestment of its responsibility of care home provision by the County Council, progresses apace. Seeing no prospect of this being altered to any worthwhile extent by group action, I chose to deal directly with its officers in writing. Their response was immediate, my suggestions and recommendations were not only agreed with, but accepted with courtesy and promise given that I would have further chance to influence the outcome.

Those words were of great help for one dares not to think of the ramifications, should any major change to my wife's lifestyle be necessary.

That said, minor happenings regarding Mary's care remain ongoing when they shouldn't be, when one takes into account the certificates of competence and the known wish of senior members of staff that this should not be. Without exception they are irritating in that they just shouldn't be happening and when certain ones recur month after month, I find myself thinking that a change of provider is perhaps the best chance of stopping them. I certainly see no point in mentioning them here in detail, but will just cite a couple, or so. The first concerns medication which should never be found left for the patient to take and certainly odd pills should not be found on the floor, within drawers, clothing and bedding, not having been taken.

The second results simply from persons not reading what is clearly printed on items, or not recording, or informing of certain happenings. The other is far more disturbing, for it is infrequent, but recurring and tears accompany the whispered revelation, along with statements about being treated harshly and thus wanting to die. Obviously I don't want to believe them, can I really believe them, and yet? If I went to the manager I know all hell would let loose, for I'm certain action would be taken, however I can't quote Mary lest it be dismissed as a product of her imagination. Thus quite naturally, only if I witness it myself will any report I make be taken as credible information, however, there is little chance of that happening. When I stress this fact to Mary, her response each time is to state the obvious in that - while I myself am around, everyone of course is on their best behaviour.

As I have said I don't want to believe what she says, yet on the other hand I'm certain she is not deliberately telling lies and there are as one might say, 'straws in the wind' to support this. Firstly there are things like the medication faults, but why is it that upon entry to her room

I sometimes find Mary left only partly dressed and that many bruises, or cut skin have never been satisfactorily explained? Why too do items have the ability to disappear from time to time? One quickly makes an assessment of peoples personalities and there are one, or two I'm suspicious of, while from the remainder about seven I would trust implicitly. The ever changing staff where very few remain long term, is another factor regarding continuity and routine implementation.

Interestingly, time has proven that Mary's judgement turns out to be the same as mine in regard to the ones I'm not happy about and one incident of derogatory sarcasm to others, was within my hearing one lunch time. This was reported in the form of a quiet word to the deputy manager, with a request that where possible the perpetrator should be placed on duties elsewhere in the building, but so far this has not entirely removed her from the scene. A subject like this should never have to be aired where care is concerned, but people are very different and despite their qualifications, like any other it's a job to which they come carrying their individual traits and the stresses and strains of the outside world.

Change of Character

    The moral compass with which the young were once equipped, in home, school and church in long passed days is sadly no longer evident, so is it any wonder that we live in such an uncaring world. To those of us old enough to have known and enjoyed a far kinder world, much could and should be different, but at the risk of being considered awkward and old fashioned, one has to amend one's criticisms. With the passing of further weeks as I have described, a completely unexpected statement one morning that someone had hit Mary, put the situation in an entirely different light and decreed that I had to take action! Requesting an appointment with the manager, I felt it best to state that I needed to get certain things clear and asked that I might submit these in writing for consideration, with a meeting later to learn what response there might be.

    This course of action being accepted, I submitted my concerns and it was indeed a worthwhile exercise, for at the meeting that ensued I was to find that the manager placed in the same position, would have done exactly the same. Our lengthy conversation was to reveal details of my wife's behaviour during the times when I was absent and this put into context her outpourings to me; so that it was not difficult to believe that the reported 'hit', had never actually taken place. Indeed as you will soon read, much was directly related to her ongoing deterioration. Somewhat painfully this fact would now be proven in my ensuing contacts with her in the visits that followed.

    To put it in a nutshell, spiteful utterances and a measure of aggression were now featuring as they had during her last months at home. Carers were now having to assist with Mary's dressing etc and, in the process, certain of them were on the receiving end of such outbursts, as she insisted that she needed no such help. Not only this, but while remonstrating with them, myself was also apparently included in her outbursts of condemnation. We were equally the cause of all her troubles!

Further complication resulted from the fact that dressing and the administering of medication could not apparently take place if the patient objected, regardless of any detrimental effect. Another use of the dreaded Health and Safety like legislation's gone wild in my view, for neither could it be insisted upon that stockings related to water retention, were worn. These short stockings and tights when worn were like other day clothing supposed to be removed at night and not left on, legs were supposed to be creamed morning and night and a footstool too should have been used while sitting, but neither could be insisted upon!

Thus are the ways of officialdom, but none of this had ever been a problem while Mary was at home, other than bathing and this quite understandable where personal privacy was concerned. In answer to my ever recurring questions relating to what to expect next in relation to her deterioration, nothing could be suggested for cases are apparently infinitely variable, other than it would only get worse! That I of course know, but at what time scale? Especially so when it is revealed that certain of the medication no longer has much effect, for that time is now passed!

Meanwhile winter has descended yet again and the dark nights and long hours confined at home accelerate my own isolation, for we are both trapped in a treadmill of recurring loneliness with unfathomable duration. This has now been exacerbated by the fact that any thought of a home visit, or even a run out into the countryside has had to be completely abandoned due to the unpredictability of her behaviour, no longer allowing me to drive safely. One aspect of this was that pleas increased for release from her 'prison', something which might be assuaged I imagined, by my spending more time with her. Thus I decided that an alternative to the weekend outing might be a longer visit, from Saturday tea time through to Sunday morning; if this was permissible.

Indeed it was, subject to knowing exact times to understandably comply with fire regulations. This accomplished, a total of four fortnightly occurring visits have now taken place. Not exactly comfortable where a single bed is concerned, but a quieter evening environment has seen return to enjoyment of DVDs such as Downton, comedy favourites and music, all surprisingly uninterrupted. As if to emphasise the 'don't count your chickens' aspect the most recent though was sadly not the case, for nothing, not even the most strenuous effort, could stop an unmitigated flow of anguished query about anything and everything for more than 4 hours, with every answer immediately forgotten in one of the most exhausting encounters of that kind.

Is the End Approaching?

In fact that's only the half of it, for it was only a few short weeks from when a photo was taken which belied the existence of any illness, but as predicted the decline has accelerated. The visits of an increased number of days too, have had to be terminated early, to leave a forlorn lost soul stood in the corridor and it has been noticeable how different many of my morning arrivals have been. No longer is there the previous excitement at my arrival and cries of joy and many more hours are filled with recriminations, regarding what I have supposedly done. Some has been so hurtful and vindictive that I can only imagine it relates to long ago happenings and living with the previous husband in particular.

Of all else, these are the most difficult to bear and time and again I am reminded of the expression 'possessed by the devil'; for all are provocative, barbed and delivered forcibly, by a soul who in truth is so gentle, loving and peaceful! This is the same face and voice which continues to express a tender love and which can apologise profusely for causing pain when I am spurred to retort - "Why Me!" It's one thing as I might have said before; to accept that memory loss and confusion are caused by fatty deposits acting as insulators that restrict minute electrical signals within the brain, but no such explanation can ever explain why there is such a profound change of character.

Special Events

Christmas and New Year have now come and gone and the situation remains little changed. Two significant occasions were to mark its passage. The first of these was for us to go on an outing to an out of town garden centre by coach, this being organised by the home. It was to be memorable in that for a few short hours, we could recapture a glimpse of times now long passed and fit briefly into life in the outside world. Upon arrival, use of her wheelchair enabled us both to commence an exploration of the many colourful and attractive items on display. Amongst its many aspects of home and garden, 'pets corner' as one of her favourites brought her pleasure and after admiring much, there was time to partake of tea and cake.

As on the previous seaside outing it was a revelation, for free of her 'prison' there were smiles, laughter and genuine enjoyment of what had so long been absent from her life. It was if a curtain had been lifted to reveal the person that I loved so desperately and who still resided within the body often so obviously inhabited by what I now term the 'Alzheimer person'. The refreshment consumed, it was now time for a last look round and opportunity to purchase one or two of the items which she had taken special interest in during the earlier walkabout. I had felt proud to wheel her around for she looked radiant in comparison to the other members of the party and so much so that again it was a case that no one else would have guessed her affliction was any more than ambulatory.

Christmas itself was to be a little special, for now unable to risk how she might react if taken home; I had asked if it might be possible for us to dine together in an upstairs meeting room on both days? Most certainly was the answer and on Christmas day itself an excellent meal came accompanied by an illuminated tree, crackers and all the trimmings. As with the recent trip out she was fine, a fact readily shown in photos of us at the feast and so, so full were we that upon retiring to her room I suggested she lay on the bed while I sat in a chair beside her. So placed we had a little doze while holding hands and with peace and tranquillity reigning, it was late evening before I took my leave, buoyed up with the thought that Boxing day might be likewise.

Sadly it was not to be and one can be so wrong in these estimations. What was provided was indeed excellent, but as the meal drew to a close, there was indication of a change of atmosphere. Trying to maintain composure, I reflected on how enjoyable the previous day had been, but on the innocent mention of the word 'bed' a torrent of anger and abuse was unleashed! Nothing I could say could pause, let alone end it and without relating further on the outburst only relatively few minutes would elapse, before I had to abdicate the encounter in despair. 'Pig sick!' is the common way of expressing it, 'Gutted' is another that says it like it is, but whatever you say the emptiness of returning home yet again to the empty house, when you hoped for so much more, was painful in the extreme.

This far down the line I can readily imagine what bereavement must feel like, but although its time span is variable, it can ultimately have an end. Alzheimer's on the other hand can suitably be described as one long, ongoing bereavement that never lets up and endlessly rubs in the loss of the loved one ad infinitum, until you despair of it ever ending.

You long for the release of your loved one from its grip, unable to contemplate what it must be like for them, you also long for the time when you don't have to witness their decline into oblivion and likewise wonder if indeed you will live long enough to see that time and if so, will you be capable of anything other than being totally exhausted in body, mind and spirit? As the calendar indicates mid-February 2012 and snow once more retards thought that Spring is just around the corner, the daily routine continues. Occasionally there will be what I call a good day, although no day can truly ever be called good in the circumstances that prevail. Better would be a more suitable adjective, for it's as ever walking on eggshells, holding your breath and hoping that it will last when it is all right and dreading those words, mother, or the former home, being mentioned as the precursor of a further debilitating encounter with the unrelenting Alzheimer's person.

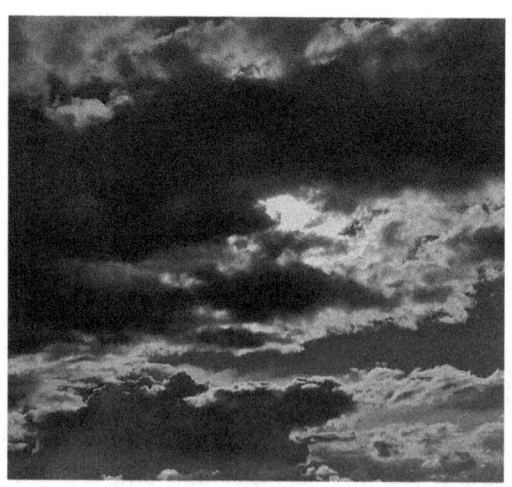

More Frustration

As at Christmas, I still have to leave before I have planned, for once commenced I have yet to discern any means to quell the outpourings, which increasingly contain abuse and accusation of what I am supposed to have done. The approach of her lunch time more often than not spells doom, for Mary is expected, quite rightly, to move to the dining area and that disruption of only relatively few feet, like someone else entering the room will render the visit unsustainable.

This said, there are still brief periods of heavenly normality, when as I have said Mary will apologise profusely for her behaviour, when I explain why she can no longer come home, or go out for a ride in the car. Where she is in her 'flat' as I term it, is of course generally good, however, this is continually and regrettably marred by the aspects that I have already referred to, regarding the niceties of her care and personal property. I recently had another talk with the manager after meeting her while on my way in one morning. Helpful and understanding as ever, I was tempted to ask her if there might be any counselling available? This was still something I felt uncomfortable about, for it patently showed my inability to cope and was thus most embarrassing.

I was really now doubting how much more I could take of what I have called these relentless mind games. Her mention of the already encountered organisation as you might guess went down as they say like a lead balloon, but my expressing this led to the suggestion that she did know someone who could help. Four weeks then went by during which time I heard nothing and as you do I chastised myself for asking, for wasn't it only really what I expected on previous experience? I was going to leave it at that, but upon encountering her again and being asked how I was, I felt bound to say I had heard nothing. "I know" she said, it didn't work out funding has been cut so I couldn't help you!

Fair enough, I don't doubt she tried, but when I look through Mary's fortnightly 'Yours' magazine, it has a regular feature on Carers and the relatives of Alzheimer's sufferers. Like various organisations publicity, it is full of stories of the help that's available; thereby giving I fear the general public a view that everything's just marvellous. It's no wonder people never ask, never offer, they doubtless believe that one has an easy life and that every need is catered for. The odd cases where it just gets too hard to bear, never feature, only sometimes does a whistle blower prompt an article in a newspaper.

Incidentals likewise occur to initially set one wondering. Things have gone missing before, but when the top of a Tupperware container relative to my taking in 'goodies', it seemed like an unlikely object to disappear; unless someone was being spiteful. A day or so earlier, I had noticed too that some writing which stated our love for each other and which had endured for some eighteen months, was now partially eradicated. Mystifying and the more so when a photograph of us both likewise then went missing from a wall. This was sufficient to speak to the deputy manager rather strongly, in terms that I had better not leave cash in my jacket whilst hung on the door, whilst being ignorant of who the culprit actually was! It prompted a more thorough search of the room while Mary was at the hairdressers and myself getting humiliated. The lid was found behind a wardrobe, the photo was found placed within newspapers about to be thrown out and upon hearing this, I knew immediately who had attempted to erase the statement proclaiming our love!

It related to my being constantly blamed of late by Mary for her 'locking up'. This was now a recurring facet of conversation day by day, along with remonstration as to my ruining everything, when she at last had a chance of happiness. A further now regular diatribe related to 'they' were looking for me, the police too being mentioned and 'they' would be stopping me visiting. She now imagines all manner of things in these confused ramblings, which are in no way regular, but increasingly worrying.

Conveying my anxieties to the deputy manager, she agreed to my request for a visit from the doctor. This duly took place and in concert with earlier ones at home, after reports from the deputy and myself, Mary's opinion was sought. She was happy, everything was fine, she felt well, there was nothing wrong with her, she could move easily and never feels faint! Thankfully, one assumes he is well used to these outpourings from dementia sufferers and this would appear to be the case, for I now learn that an appraisal is to be made by a doctor from another source.

It's a wonderful feeling though when you do know that someone cares and indeed I would shortly find that someone did, due to some niggling health issues. A couple of these which had never really been adequately dealt with by my doctor, finally prompted me to consult another. This done, not only did he put in place the means by which these might be rectified, but took time to inquire how I was coping stress wise. When informed that things were becoming increasingly difficult and that I was wilting under the pressure, he first offered medication. This I declined, for dulling the senses answers nothing, it's a friend you need, someone to talk to, someone who's very being there will lift your spirits. To his great credit, what he said next brought me great comfort, for if I found it getting too much for me I should make an appointment to see him, solely to talk things out. As post mortem as one might say, rather than being instantly available, it nevertheless was greatly appreciated. In contrast, what was to follow elsewhere was completely unexpected and most demoralising.

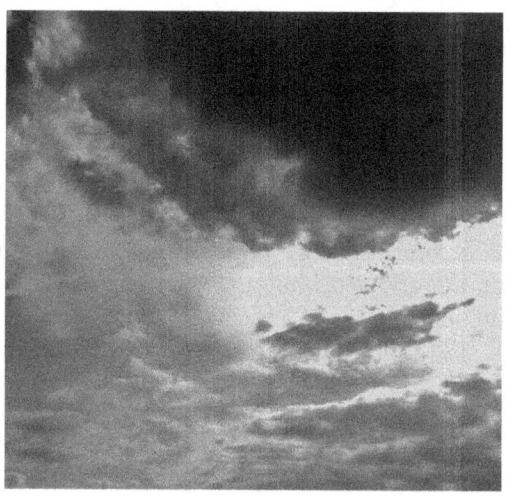

Threats and Intimidation

Many weeks had passed since the last occasion when I had stayed with Mary at the home overnight. That single bed wasn't very comfortable and the subject, somewhat to my relief, had not since been mentioned. Notwithstanding this fact, one, or two better daytime visits would produce the request that I again stay. It wasn't forgotten as I had hoped, so the next Saturday morning I arrived well stocked with DVDs to firstly see how the day would go. In fact it went remarkably well, frighteningly well like no other and the euphoria lasted throughout the evening until around 9 o'clock, when it was requested she take her night time medication.

This she would not do and I prepared to leave. Not even the threat of this was sufficient to get them administered, so the Carer left the room. Once she departed peace again reigned, for of course her entry, like those where there is enquiry as to the lunch time menu, provokes a mood change. With quiet resumed I decided to stay after all, wishing all the time that the Carer had left the pills with me to administer. It was destined to be my last night as it happened, for peaceful as it was and continued thus through washing, dressing, breakfast and my departure; however once I had left, things apparently changed substantially.

Knowing nothing of this, I was somewhat mystified by a call requesting my meeting the manager. This being arranged, I attended still unaware of what the reason might be, but soon found out in no uncertain terms. This was not the face of the previously known caring manager, but that resembling the much earlier Social Services 'Starsi'. "This must not happen again, it cannot be tolerated, medication must be given and I can't have my staff putting up with difficult residents!" Shocked; was I? You bet, but agreed to cease night visits, asking that it not be a dramatic end for my wife's sake, should she query it.

"It must end now else she could stay there no longer and the alternative was a mental home and (almost in spite), she wouldn't like that, for it would be noisy!" How did I feel on hearing this outburst? Shafted! is the best description. It took a while for it to sink in. What about those previous statements that we can't make the patients take their medication, it's their decision. What happened to the care aspect? Weren't these supposed to be Carers trained to deal with behaviour change and if they couldn't cope with this; how to God would they have coped as I had, with month after month of aggravation 24/7 and trapped within four walls with no training, or assistance whatever!

Needless to say conversation (if there is any), with that person will be restricted to the barest minimum from now on and I remain shocked that I should be subjected to her outburst in the first place. It wasn't the only unpleasant encounter either, for as you will have read all rides out had been stopped, for the simple fact that you can't drive a vehicle with an agitated and disturbed passenger. The answer if it were possible was to find someone Mary knew and liked to travel with us as distraction. Initially that person also needed to drive, for one of my health problems was foot related. At the home Mary got on famously with one person, who visited in some kind of helper role.

It seemed I might have found the solution and should she be willing was ready to reimburse her. However, when I saw her and put the question her response was entirely negative, stating insurance considerations as the reason. Fair enough, but I was disappointed for she seemed the ideal person. I had previously mentioned my desire to arrange something of this nature to the manager, to counter Mary's pleas regarding being locked in and she knew that I would ask that person again, now that my foot improvement meant that I could do the driving. (I ask that you again remember that bit.)

After the passing of several weeks, I encountered this person who was normally so kindly and began the conversation, by saying I understood her reason for declining. "No! No!" she almost shouted. "Hang on", I said "I haven't said anything yet! "No! No! No! so I gave up. In the hours that followed, I noted that she deliberately ignored Mary during the several times that she passed us during that day. The reason for her behaviour? Your guess is as good as mine, but I think I have a clue.

A little while later I was told that such institutions have a non-fraternisation clause in the contracts of their employees, so if this is so and the woman is bound by it; why couldn't she have been more forthcoming in the first instance and why so rude? Also as I have said the manager knew what I would be asking, so why on earth not explain the situation, then I wouldn't have asked any further! Indeed it would not be the last time that that attitude was displayed. At times I despair, for so many little signs are there all the time to question the level of care. Days still go by where no water is available in the room and yesterday a plate with breakfast remnants was still unmoved when I left mid-afternoon. Likewise today another pill was found at bedside, after what I had felt was a reliable dispenser had been the one to administer it. Where she was concerned I encountered a further dearth of care as follows, after the day had started beautifully, with Mary happy and content.

It lasted for just two hours, or more until like many others, the spell was broken by someone entering the room to ask what she would like for lunch. From then until around two thirty confusion reigned within Mary's head and that Carer knowing the situation, was asked twice if she might arrange a cup of tea as palliative. Yes was her answer, with the promise she would return, but needless to say nothing was done. Two to three months having passed as you will now read, things are little better. Mary's slow deterioration has continued apace, with there being much less opportunity to enjoy anything but short periods of music, film, or conversation.

Mobility was also deteriorating, so that short walks within the confines of the building were restricted and those that did take place were much shorter. A definite surprise was that a totally unexpected ride out was possible one morning, when a surplus of staff, allowed one of them to accompany us. Confining its duration somewhat, I took a well-known route, but soon realised that Mary showed almost no recognition of any of the places passed along the way. This loss of memory aspect of her affliction I am by now well aware of, but nevertheless I am daily astounded by its totality! I find myself reminded of something in the Bible, some words of Jesus - "I am". If I understand it correctly he meant his existence was endless, unbounded and as such was reassuring and comforting.

Double Standards

Mary's condition on the other hand is beyond my comprehension, for having only very limited early memories and current retention only of two minutes maximum, "I am" present tense only; perhaps best describes her existence! What on earth must it be like for her? The nearest I can think of is being lost on moor land in a thick fog, unable to see what's behind, to either side, or in front, but knowing that you do at least exist! I choose that example, for I experienced it around 55 years ago when travelling between Buxton and Macclesfield via the well-known Cat and Fiddle route.

Roads, nor their signing, were as good then and thick fog in the darkness of an early Autumn evening, somehow saw me take a minor road on one of the many tight turns that abound. In no time at all the road petered out and when the vehicle was exited, no clue was there of reality. One might as well have been suddenly dumped on a foreign planet! The word lost doesn't adequately describe it and that must be how Mary now feels. Provided regularly with the essentials, my visits must seem to equate to the arrival of a guide for a few hours, so no wonder she pleads with me so often not to leave her and stresses how alone she feels; just as I did that dark night long years ago. I suggest this might be a good time to stop for a moment, or two and attempt yourself to imagine it.

Returning to the ride out, it was interesting from another point of view, for this time there was no mention of any of the oft quoted, supposed insurance restrictions, regarding my being accompanied by a member of staff while they were on duty. This too was the case more recently, when I drove Mary to hospital for a brain scan. This came about following my request for her doctor to carry out a reappraisal of her medication, something that resulted from my concern that over a long period; she had complained almost daily of dizziness and weakness.

The hospital trip couldn't have gone better in fact and came within a period during which more ticks than crosses appeared on my calendar, as a measure of how pleasant my recent visits to the home had been. Of course there were bad days when I had to leave early and as ever, often everything would have gone well until there was some interruption, to precipitate a rapid change of mood. If Mary was feeling sleepy, I found it profitable to encourage her to take a nap and by this means any confrontational aspects were either prevented, or at least delayed. Indeed perhaps things were going a little too smoothly, but only a week later I took a phone call early one morning, that brought great concern about Mary's care and confrontation was the product.

JOHN ENGLAND

An Unsolved Mystery

I was advised that Mary had had a fall, had cut her leg and had been taken to hospital. It didn't quite make sense. I couldn't imagine anywhere in her room, that had anything capable of cutting a leg, but without hesitation made my way to the hospital and enquired as to in which ward might she be found? Directed to A & E, it was suggested I go down a corridor which I knew led to where the ambulances arrive. A nurse who I met asked where I was going. When I explained, she replied "Oh it's you, follow me." Taken to one of the receiving rooms, I was to find Mary being attended to by a doctor and a nurse, who were attempting to remove bandages and clean up the substantial amount of blood, from the large slice which had been cut from Mary's leg.

They, no more than I, could readily understand how it happened, but proceeded to complete a somewhat lengthy rebuilding of the torn tissues. It looked nasty and although I was told she had had the strongest pain relieving injection, I could see Mary remained in great pain. Interestingly I was allowed to watch, as between them they commenced what I can only describe as 'a beautiful bit of surgery'. Their task comprised stitching within the body of the leg, ahead of replacing a hanging flap of flesh which without exaggeration measured around 8 x 2½ inches and sewing it into place. Bearing in mind the severity of this wound, they like myself could not believe it was consistent with a fall in her room.

Their work done, Mary and I were left alone while arrangements were made to return her to the home. She didn't want anything to eat, but the tea that was provided was very welcome and after we had chatted for some twenty five minutes, she appeared to doze off, however, something didn't seem right and my first reaction was to suspect it was the shock of the operation, that had recently been completed. As the minutes mounted, my attempt to wake her failed and I contemplated pulling an alarm cord, but hesitated in fear of being made to look foolish. I knew Mary was alive, for her breathing continued, although it was somewhat laboured but eventually I resorted to pulling the cord. It seemed an age before anyone came, but on seeing the situation the nurse cancelled any thought of returning to the Home and transfer was arranged to a reception ward for tests.

Questionable Care

It was good that I was there, for both nurses, doctor and a consultant had many questions to be answered relating to there being any previous occurrences and as you may well remember they were very isolated and went back some four, or more years. The hospital conclusion was that they were seizures, or fits and I encountered the word epilepsy as a new aspect of Mary's condition. Yet another pill was thus added to her daily intake and its minimal dose would initially seem to be successful. However, before I relate further on this, I must backtrack somewhat, to relate further on the twists and turns of the care aspect.

Questions certainly remain in my mind as to this and if the leg wound relates to it. The abysmal 2012 weather meant that my weekend visits increased and as I have already said, my arrival was in early morning when care is almost non-existent. Thus on many days I had arrived to find the unit bereft of anyone, for when the residents are being got up, washed and dressed etc, the term 'going behind closed doors' is used. Fine if there's another to watch over the other five inmates, but unfortunately that was not often the case. If an alarm is triggered by say someone getting out of bed, there was a chance that someone would come up from downstairs, but they have their own work to do, are slow to arrive and understandably promptly return thence.

On the day in question I was told that a Carer 'behind closed doors' heard the alarm activated as my wife got out of bed and as soon as practical, looked out in the corridor to find my wife fallen in her doorway and then realising the situation was acute, called for assistance. At the hospital, I was asked several times as to how much blood was lost, something which I did not know. Subsequently, the Home's management said it was very little, however privately I was told it was a large amount and that concurs with what I saw as the bandages were removed. At a complete loss to imagine how such a major wound could be obtained, it has since been suggested that during the fall my wife must have turned 180 degrees, for the footrests of her wheelchair to be the cause of cutting into her right leg.

However, I could find no trace of blood whatever upon them, their surfaces remaining in an 'as new' condition. I've said before that when Mary says something about what goes on while I'm not there, experience and investigation proves that what she has said is indeed founded on fact, such as being dealt with by a previously unknown Carer. Only last week I arrived early one morning to find her the only sign of life, wandering the empty corridor repeating over and over - "Oh God please help me." On another morning I could hear that she was very unhappy about something, before I was anywhere near her room.

Immediately I entered the room it was clear to see why. Sat on a chair she was only partly dressed and her toilet had discarded night wear on the floor. I knew that someone had recently been around, for a mug of tea was still hot, but why on earth was she left like this, for I had now realised her underclothes were soaking! Yet again no one was to be found, but a green light signified that a Carer was 'behind closed doors' and she remained thus for some time. When she eventually emerged I found it to be one whom I trusted and who I thought might now throw some light on my findings. How wrong was I in this regard; for every attempt I made to speak to her was met with a barrage of, "I know nothing, I was behind closed doors"!

It was persistent and could be likened to a game of 'snap', when 'snap' is called before each card even leaves your hand. It was ridiculous and when five, or six attempts to speak brought only this theatrical response, I began to get angry. It developed into a shouting match and when I finally got a word in after twice threatening to report her to management; she finally quietened down, enabling me to ask her if she knew anything that might throw light on what I had found. Again it was a case of a Carer from downstairs responding to an alarm, making the tea and then leaving. All else like so much more, has to be left to pure speculation!

No speculation whatever was, however, required on a more recent happening though, rather confirmation and this from an outside source; namely the district nurses visiting regularly to treat Mary's leg wound. Having changed the method of dressings to speed what looked to be a very long treatment period, they made it known that a compression stocking was to be worn all the time. Needless to say it wasn't, despite being entered in the diary and it was obvious that they were not at all pleased.

Nor was I, on another aspect of care, indeed a constantly recurring one, that of Mary having nothing to drink, even though it is supposed to be a legal requirement as I understand. It happened on both the Monday and Tuesday, with there also being no breakfast on Monday! I am aware of this because I was there both days and know it was twice promised as was something to drink; however nothing ever came. As you know I had made such shortcomings known long ago, but such things continue without being remedied. That said, by Wednesday I was prompted to speak out somewhat vigorously as you are about to learn. With the hospital initially deciding on a low dose pill to counter the epilepsy, it was reasonable to expect they would want to see Mary back at the hospital as a follow up procedure.

Having read this far into this book you may, by now, be wondering why I had not seen fit to place Mary's name beneath a Dedication at its beginning. Indeed this was suggested but I declined for, in revealing so much, it would already be obvious she was the prime candidate for that honour. Quiet and unassuming, Mary was the last person to want publicity and perhaps, at first, might not have liked the idea of this publication but would, nevertheless, wholeheartedly accept the fact that this could be the means towards some very necessary changes. This being so and, in particular, with the ever-widening reach of this disease, the most fitting Dedication here should certainly be:

'To all Family Carers'

Yet More Confrontation

With this visit now imminent, my expectation was that the successful visit procedure of a few weeks back would be repeated and I would take both she and the Carer to the appointment in my car. Not so, for again this supposed special insurance matter was quoted as to why I would not. Getting a little tired of this prevarication, I decided to ring my own insurers to see what they thought. As I guessed it made no sense at all to them whatever and it was suggested that the Home should ring the insurers and provide some believable explanation. Sure that this would end what I took to be a farcical situation, it was however never resolved, for the Home had other ideas.

On Wednesday I was informed that "it would be in my wife's best interest", for her to travel to the hospital with the Carer, therefore I was not required. I was insulted by this and the tone of the edict was similar to the earlier encounter with regard to overnight stays. I bided my time, but when I later left the building, I saw the office door open and expressed myself forcibly, addressing this Mrs 'best decision' without any ceremony, or respect. I was not pleased and let her know it. She replied that those best interests were based on the facts that it was thought I looked ill and should my wife distract me, I wouldn't be capable of driving safely. This was sheer unadulterated b****cks and my response was as follows.

If Mary's 'best interests' were so important, it was a pity that the nurses instructions weren't followed; rather than they have to take their disquiet to the manager. Also was it in her 'best interests' to not have any breakfast on

Monday and also have nothing to drink all day on either Monday, or Tuesday! I reminded her that I had brought this matter up before and that this insurance business made no sense whatsoever, when only a few weeks back I had carried a member of staff on not one, but two occasions! Her response was to insist on her decision and by chance the manager entered the room in time to hear of the risk of dehydration. She agreed there was a case to answer and after I left I would have just loved to have been a fly on the wall.

Suffice to say the next three visits were hydrated as never before and during the most recent we were offered tea no less than five times and at midday the jug of water was replaced with one of cordial! As for the driving ban, it was expected that I would make my own way to the hospital and meet them on their arrival, but I would not and said this emphatically. Much as I would have loved to be by Mary's side, I don't dance to the snap of someone else's fingers. I had been classed as 'only her husband' and it hurt. On too many occasions this 'officialdom knows best' is proclaimed. They think they know it all, but don't and never will and one is left feeling it's a pity the purveyor of these edicts don't have a mother, father, or husband so afflicted; for only then will they really know what it's like at the sharp end!

Anyway there's an old saying that one should never attempt to come between man and wife and I remain convinced, that there would have been times when my recollection of the various episodes of Mary passing out over a four year period, plus the latest whilst in A & E would have been of use, had I have been present at the Hospital. As I'm sure I've already said, over a substantial number of Hospital and Surgery visits spanning many years; I had been Mary's proxy memory. Over all I had given doctors and consultants the information they required and not only been thanked by them, but indeed commended; in that this fact demonstrated an unusual care and devotion. It is now early November 2012 as the saga is related further and the leg wound is healing nicely, due to the regular and highly professional visits by District Nurses. Only yesterday, I read that the totally necessary and excellent service they provide is to be hit by spending cuts, while administrative position salaries in the NHS and elsewhere pursue the entirely opposite direction!

As far as Mary is concerned her decline now again exhibits, what seems like some small improvement. Although she often asks why she can't come home, there is now more quiet acceptance and less difficulty regarding her ever stated need to visit her Mother. Of late, my saying these are 'old' memories that persist, rather than today's, more often than not brings this subject to a peaceful conclusion. Of course it hasn't all been honey, for several weeks I wasn't able to stay till lunch time, or even earlier.

On those occasions at around mid-day I had to go, either because I was told it was time I went, or it was because 'her husband' was expected. I learnt long ago to take it as it comes. To be thankful if it's been a good day and to try to look forward rather than be miserable if it's bad; for tomorrow it might be all the better. One thing above all, I try my utmost to leave expressing my undying love. Mary too, is far frailer now and the reduction in her mobility over the last four to five months is very pronounced. It means she is unable to complete our walks along the corridors and so much so that some twenty five feet is now her maximum.

The falls too continue mainly either within, or upon leaving her en suite facilities. Often they are related to what I term panic attacks, where she is suddenly transfixed, unable to move, before sinking to the floor. Where this is concerned I had been told to summon help ahead of any toilet need, for it has been found that if a Carer is present there seems less chance that Mary will get into difficulty due to simply 'giving up'. This 'sympathetic' aspect of vulnerability and the demand for close attendance, likewise manifests itself most afternoons, when I am inveigled into delaying my departure, by unending reminder regarding her loneliness.

True Mary is lonely, but I am too in an unforgiving empty house, which now that Winter is upon us is a far less acceptable option to the warmth and comfort she enjoys, not to say security. My guessing that the panic attacks were more likely to be linked to the epilepsy aspect was later confirmed with dramatic effect as December arrived, heralding a whole new gut wrenching aspect, of what by now had become a four and a half year struggle with the affliction of dementia.

Prologue to Disaster

Over previous weeks those panic attacks had continued, sometimes requiring one, or more helper plus a hoist, to regain normality. Notwithstanding, plans had been made so that as at last Christmas we could dine together, watch DVDs, listen to favourite music and enjoy surroundings that were as near as possible to our home. That is, until one particular Tuesday visit. Somewhat difficult from the start, when the toilet was required, Mary found it impossible to stand. With a Carer called as incentive it was no different, so in an attempt to get her thence a wheeled chair was brought. Transferred with difficulty to this, it was pulled backwards towards the toilet, however she suddenly struck out, limbs stiffened and eyes glazed over to provide an unforgettable impression of hugely, non-understood behaviour.

Eventually this passed, but by the time she had been returned to her chair, I was too shaken to want to remain any longer. Did I but know it, it would be the last time I would be with her in that room, once recovered, as ever she didn't want me to leave and believe it, or not after all that frightening 'performance' Mary followed me all the way down the corridor to the door walking boldly without hesitation. She was perfectly upright as she hadn't been for months and presumably returned to her room in the same manner!

Towards noon next day, I was to receive a phone call. A doctor who had been called, had decided to send Mary to hospital and that I should await instruction as to when she might arrive there. With memory of the recent leg episode in A & E, I decided to make my way there at once. However, I then found it impossible to advise the home of this fact. Finding her not yet arrived, I was told to wait in the day room until advised and did so for a full two hours. Imagining I had been forgotten, I made enquiry and found she had yet to arrive and neither could any time be given when this might be! My wait finally ended some six or more hours after the ambulance had been called. An ambulance man who directed me to her, said Mary had been talking to him on the way from the home, but I was to find her in the reception area, wild eyed, with unintelligible speech and intermittent and wildly flailing legs.

For over two hours, under repeated promise that nurse would return, or a doctor arrive "in a minute", I was left without aid, or information, with the hopeless task of trying to stop the often flailing legs. Those same legs that had so recently been restored to health by painstaking care, were despite my best efforts, being relentlessly bruised and battered anew. That cubicle in essence recreated those four walls in which I had been powerless to temper the circumstances at home for more than two years and something had to be done!

On the wall was a red button, so I decided to activate it. It certainly did the trick, for we were immediately descended upon by what seemed around 20 persons, 'from out of the woodwork', as they say and were they animated! Prominent among these very alarmed ones was the nurse who had kept us waiting and she was angry, for I had done something very wrong! - But how was I to know it was the cardiac arrest alarm! I had had enough and wasn't going to take that lying down.

I pursued her for some distance, stating the endless promises and loudly declared that should something not be done; they had better realise they would need to arrange another bed for me! These words resulted in the prompt appearance of a doctor, who after only the briefest of contact, said he needed to check some blood results. And, would you believe it - "He would be back in a minute"! Another forty minutes though elapsed before his return and by then a fiasco that had lasted since before noon was unresolved as 9pm approached. As politely as I could, but very firmly, I said I had really had enough, I was going home and the responsibility was all his.

There are times when you think it just can't get any worse, but believe me it can and for the next 30 plus days it did and increasingly so, so prepare yourself. Those of you with no experience of Dementia will have already read much of the preceding pages with disbelief, but others whose family has been touched, will by reading on, start thanking God very substantially that their particular experience ended before it got this far. As such it would have primarily been a supreme blessing to their loved one, but also would have deprived them of some truths of today's society that are better left unknown.

That aspect though comes a little later and shattered as I was by the previous day's experience, I now sought the assistance of a neighbour as escort, in my return to the hospital next morning to find Mary. At something after 9am I was to find her in a ward looking absolutely pathetic, best expressed as out for the count; totally unresponsive and but a shadow of even the previous day, awful as that was. There was no point of staying as I saw it so I returned home, pausing at the desk to request that I be advised as soon as she might be restored to any normality.

Note - This was readily agreed by not one, but two persons also on duty, for as she looked my greatest trauma existed in the fact that should the worst scenario transpire, there had been no chance whatsoever to say a Good-bye. As the hours slowly passed it was this thought that was uppermost in my mind. I could only endure and wait, wait for that telephone call, else it would haunt me for the rest of my life. So, so many days, endless days had previously passed in fact, when I had waved, blown that last kiss and turned away, wondering if it had in fact been out last meeting here on earth.

As each hour passed it emphasised the agony of not knowing and the tears began to flow as never before. At around 1pm, I had to talk to someone and rang the home after some difficulty finding myself connected to the manager, who had been cut off in the middle of a conversation with another. Explaining the situation she commiserated, urging that I try to remember the many good times, for she likewise felt the continued silence was at the very least ominous.

Two hours later I rang the neighbour to ask if he would accompany me once more at around 7.30pm, so that I might say my last good-bye to the supposed inert figure, which could surely not remain so till another morning. He promptly agreed and for me, the time had come to truly learn what the loss of a loved one actually feels like. Around two further distressing hours were to pass to compile the agony, then the phone rang, it was the home's manager. She, sharing my fears, had rung the hospital to be told Mary was fine! From around half an hour after I had left she had been sitting up talking, had enjoyed her lunch and to all intents had very little wrong with her! My joy was immense, yet I was very angry that I should needlessly have been put through such pain and lost those hours of being at her side. I immediately returned to the hospital desk and stood waiting, straight away noticing that the piece of paper relating to my being informed lay in clear view of the person before me.

Eventually she asked what I wanted? Stating the anguish that I had suffered I inquired why the instruction directly in front of her had been ignored? Her curt response was, "We don't pass messages for people"! (Something else to remember a little later on in this tale.) Mary was indeed fine and my telling a member of staff that I was prepared to assist in the giving of food and medication, ensured no limit to my visits after 1030 hours. Unknowingly my ready acceptance was in time to become something of a chore, but it would reveal much that was wrong in regard to a dementia patient being placed in anything other than a specially designated ward. Mary was indeed fine, as photographs I took would prove and not only that, in similar vein to when she had first been taken into care, the Alzheimer's appeared to have gone into regression.

Said to only have a water infection, after two days the hospital naturally wished to discharge Mary back to the care home. This moment in time is where it all went wrong and the progression of decisions now encountered was unbelievable and it had all started with that doctor. To my surprise, I was told that the home's manager would need to visit to assess if Mary could return! It was a bolt from the blue I can tell you, for I had been assured on numerous occasions that Mary could continue at the home until the end. As it happened, the manager arrived for the assessment within only minutes of the hospital doctor confirming only a water infection was present and that therefore repatriation should occur. However the manager after only a perfunctory word, stated rather loudly and abruptly, "You know very well, we only do one to one not two to one"! Somewhat taken aback by this and momentarily lost for words, I could only suggest she had better talk to the doctor. This she presumably did, but did not return and through to the next morning I knew nothing of what lay before us.

Upon my entry to the ward next morning the anxiety must have shown, for a nurse asked, was I alright? On my reply of "No" and explaining why; she kindly said she would find out. A short time later, she confirmed the manager of the home had refused to take Mary back and to my asking as to what came next, she suggested that Social Services would be contacting me. That did me a lot of good for sure, for they remember, had proved to be as useful as a chocolate teapot some two and a half years previous. (Later information I have received, is that hospitalisation is often a convenient path for care homes, as it provides an opportunity to unload their clients against having to cope with increasing decline of faculties.)

This may be, but the severity of that manager's words and her non return to explain further the previous afternoon, was yet further confirmation of her ability to change in a moment, from supposed friendship to vicious self-preservation. It had happened once or twice before remember and with cruel intent when staying overnight was abruptly terminated. Now in this rejection, she had originated a progression of events that were to kill Mary and she might as well have put a gun to Mary's head in that moment. If only she had been reasonable, she could have been told of the very evident remission of the Alzheimer's, which had occurred with the change of location.

Sadly, the hospitalisation therefore had to continue and Mary now assumed the role of a bed blocker. For its part the hospital undertook an attempt to secure additional NHS funding for continuing care, for I was told nursing care was now appropriate and I digested some four pages of locations in the County offering care of various types including that for Dementia. When Mary had originally been taken into care I had needed to do nothing, it all being done by the local authority, but this time things had changed. All homes were now in private hands and there was a significant paragraph at the top of page one.

This emphasised this in its warning in BOLD type, that before making contact one should ascertain that they are prepared to accept a Social Care Contract. For my part I now unexpectedly had to attempt to find a new home for Mary, with only those sheets of paper from Social Services to guide me. So now take note of those three words - Social Care Contract. Like me you probably won't have encountered them before, but you may do yet so be prepared. In short it defines an 'us' and 'them' situation, where if like Mary and I you were in at the start in 1946 when the NHS started, care was from the Cradle to the Grave.

Not now it ain't, we're not all equal anymore; some are much more equal than others. These three words were destined to prolong Mary's time in hospital considerably and this revealed that in occupying a bed she was let us say an unnecessary inconvenience. Where medication was concerned for instance, it was found to be somewhat farcical. During what turned out to be day long visits for more than five weeks; only a few pills were seen to be given. If they were refused they were left untaken on the trolley and others were to be regularly found on the floor. Also things like eye drops which I could administer were locked away, for medication had to be locked up I was told and yet a dozen or so cards containing Mary's month's supply (at a guess several hundreds of pills), remained on the locker top, simply because the pack was too big to fit in the cabinet! Double speak for certain and there would be much more of this later.

Not wishing to be put off at an initial phone inquiry, I decided to visit a major known care provider's premises. Plush too it was at entry, I was offered refreshment, provided with a glossy brochure and interviewed by a lady of some seniority. It did she said accept a Social Care Contract and I was then led away from the plush entry, through corridors and pathways to a bungalow type building by a cheerful young woman. Code locks gave entry to a dismal corridor of cell like doors and sight of the first shuffling male inmate with a huge sn** overlapping his upper lip.

As the tour progressed, open doors revealed scruffy surroundings, unmade beds and an absence of all that Mary had enjoyed before. The change from what I could call home, or hotel like surroundings was breathtaking! The communal area had all that one might associate with an old time asylum and indeed those witnessed therein fitted that same picture. A room shown had nothing to recommend it and I'm not even sure that it even had a window. Toilets were communal rather than en suite and it was easy to imagine their condition and how someone with only a modicum of decency would be offended by them.

However it was the overriding stench throughout the building that made me want to throw up! It wasn't the expected urine either, but more an air of depravity and abandonment. Once out in the fresh air I bid farewell, saying I would be in touch, but the most pertinent thought was that if these poor creatures had anyone, anywhere that cared about them; it wouldn't be like that. In truth they must really be abandoned souls. I was shocked at what I had found, but resolved to try again for surely they couldn't all be like this, or could they?

At the second location my heart dropped, for as I entered it displayed the same logo as the first. All went reasonably well throughout the preamble of my needs and what might be available, until it came to my being shown round and the man enquired loudly across to the receptionist; "What rooms might be available under the Social Care Contract?" As I by then suspected, it was another bungalow style building with similar entry routine. At least it didn't smell as the other did and the general air of the place was a little more reasonable, but again it was dull, dingy and again had communal toilets.

On the way to it we had passed another similar building with not only plenty of windows, but also very normal care home facilities, such as a large lounge with groups of pensioners at ease in their armchairs. Where I was taken though still had the air of an asylum, its rooms still resembled cells and no more than an empty one I was shown. Scruffy and airless I still doubt any window and across the corridor there was the constant bellowing sounds as if a bull was being castrated! When I remarked upon this, for truly you couldn't hear yourself think; I was told it was only old so and so, as if it mattered not. It certainly did matter and I remarked that my wife wouldn't like it at all! Oh well, I'd better take you to a quieter part of the building, was the response.

Cap in Hand

It was I must say a little better than my first encounter with the Private sector, but in no way the place you would send a loved one, not even the most miserable old sod you can imagine. Dogs fare better, criminals in prison fare very much better and such deprivation I could no way countenance for Mary. So It was a case of two down and few to go and needless to say I had great doubt as to where all this might end. I certainly took no pleasure in going cap in hand like a pauper and this should not be, for who in truth has around £1,200 to £1,400 a week to fork out week after week? Even those who had retired from business, or who had substantial homes, would find their reserves severely depleted in very few months at that rate.

Several plush, newly built care homes all advertised vacancies, however I didn't fancy being shown the door, so initially balked at applying to those, but finally had to swallow my pride out of necessity. At about this time Mary's appetite was picking up and with ear piece loudspeakers my daily visits to hospital were able to provide her favourite music on CD and DVD, without disturbance to other patients. It too though was around this time that a male visitor coughed loudly throughout his day long visit. Why he wasn't told to leave I can't imagine, but it would prove to be something that would now put Mary's life in grave danger.

Anyway why should I flinch from approaching a new state of the art care provider? For all their pretence I knew I was better than they were. I owed no one and all I owned was through hard graft, while some of them: including the best known names, owed hundreds of millions. It's something I've never understood about 'great' companies, how they can owe these great sums and yet never go out of business. I've only ever bought what I could afford, under the old precept of income six pence; out goings five pence three farthings equals happiness! So next day I went boldly through the door of one and said as firmly as I could, "Do you accept a Social Care Contract?" "Well er", said the chap, "why don't you come and sit down, let me take a few details."

A Cook's tour was declined while refreshment was taken and copious detail given for between 20 and 30 minutes, while my original question remained unanswered. Hang on I said, I'm wasting my time, you haven't yet given an answer to what I asked. Do you accept people under the Social Care Contract? Well, yes we do have some people. Well how many? A few. Well might you accept my wife? What a palaver, I thought, but he did reveal that an assessment would be needed. Right then I said, I'm asking you to please make one and with that I left, expecting it would merely provide time to engineer a reason for rejection.

I felt at least I'd got somewhere, but I wasn't convinced, so I ventured a visit to the one other location that was reasonably easy to get to. It was located down a narrow country lane and upon arrival I rang the bell. As soon as I was invited through the door I felt a great deal better. The ambience was palpable, I felt at home, for the very woodwork conveyed peace and tranquility. There was kindness in my greeting and an eagerness to show me around, while listening to what I had to say. I was convinced right away that this was where I wanted Mary to be. Everywhere was clean and bright, each room was en suite, furniture, bed linen and curtains were stylish and large windows looked out onto lovely countryside.

I told of where I had already been and what I had found, hiding nothing and stating how I was now convinced my search had ended with what I thought was just what I wanted for Mary. In fact it was, but I wasn't to know that for another two to three weeks, during which time a cough which Mary would pick up from that hospital visitor would get worse and worse. While mine would respond to antibiotics, Mary's chest developed a harsh rattle, which would certainly do nothing towards her being accepted anywhere at all. The seemingly endless days dragged by as I treaded water as it were, while trapped by the system.

With my spending the bulk of each day by Mary's side in hospital nothing was getting done at home, other than my preparing a rushed meal each evening. The application for NHS continuing care was apparently rejected and the effect of the continued incarceration and growing infection was becoming very evident. Mary's appetite dwindled. Food and drink would not be accepted, even though I persisted. By now, Christmas and New Year had also passed when it was my turn to succumb to the chest infection, losing several valuable days, just when I needed to be by her side and to remain active where any chance of her ever being moved were concerned.

Without a zimmer Mary's mobility was now restricted to her bed and chair, for even if she could remember how to use the call button, time proved that wait could amount to fifteen, or more minutes. Thus she was placed in immense padding and soon became doubly incontinent. As the days passed her visage too deteriorated so much, that Mary was barely recognisable to that of only a fortnight earlier. Except that is, on one of two days when I wasn't there and another lady was kind enough to take my place. On this day Mary had been quite talkative and had surprised this lady, by saying that she remembered that on the day we were married, she had arrived at the church on her bike!

On the other afternoon when a zimmer was available, Mary had walked around the ward talking and with attendance had even visited the toilet. Early one evening a representative from the posh new home did actually visit to make an assessment, but I felt sure this would prove to be unfruitful. With more than a week now elapsed since the attendance of the man from the posh home, I thought it wise to enquire if any decision had been made? The question could not be answered, someone would ring back, but never did.

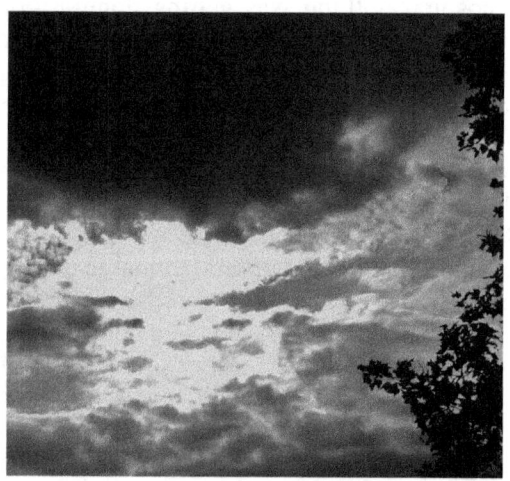

Insult to Injury

Next day I tried again and after a very long wait, received the verdict and this mind you, from a company professing to have the greatest of expertise in Dementia care. The decision had been made and my wife could not be accepted. I asked if I might be given the reason? Yes, I was told; they couldn't have her disturbing their other guests! You might be able to guess my feelings! Devastated wasn't the word for it. A couple of days later still no response was forthcoming as to what was happening, so I called the hospital requesting that the Matron please advise me, for time was ebbing away.

When I had recovered sufficiently to get to the hospital and see her, she explained that she had felt no need to ring me, for Social Services had told her I had received a full update! This was certainly not the case, for true to their reputation and my experience, the one brief contact I had had, was the presentation of the list of care homes and nothing else. Entirely unbeknown to me there was now a lifeline, for a representative from the spot in the country had by now also carried out an assessment and was willing to take Mary; except that everything still awaited a decision on funding.

This at last was good news, however, my feeling was that it was all too late, for Mary was by now looking an extremely different person to even a week earlier and it was almost impossible to communicate with her. Matron had I found, completed all the lengthy paperwork and sent it off to the PCT on the day previous, however she was now advised this had been 'Lost'. As if that wasn't enough, my resumption of visits to Mary revealed something else. Seeking to grip her hand, while gently massaging her arm to remind her of my feelings, I noticed that her finger was without our wedding ring. Along with another of her mother's that she valued greatly they had long been so tight as to defy removal, but someone it seemed had persuaded the most modern and attractive one off the finger.

When I reported this, I was told it must have simply been collected in the folds of the bedding when it was changed. What then were the chances of its recovery I asked, was it an on-site laundry? The answer of it being one in an adjacent county did nothing to assuage my feeling of loss, for it is the third such case that I am aware of and methinks it's a nice little earner that one can do very little about, bearing in mind the ever rising value of gold. It was all too coincidental. I'm sure it must have been taken by someone who knew that after all those weeks Mary would be departing, for bed linen had seen regular change, especially in regard to the onset of the incontinence.

Indeed that day's events encapsulated all that was wrong with Mary ever being sent to hospital in the first place. As in every sphere of life it was down to individuals and their incompetence. One could wait twenty minutes for response to a call button and asking was no guarantee of more alacrity in a need being met. Changing was one such function which often engendered reluctance to complete it. On one day in particular and despite my asking ahead of lunch, Mary went right through till after supper (7pm), before she was changed and here I would ask you remember the earlier remark, that 'We don't take messages'. That day in particular they certainly had done and regularly, continually back and forth because someone couldn't get through on their mobile, also a lengthy search was made to find someone an extra pillow from an adjoining ward and no expense was spared time wise, to obtain a glass of water for another person.

Discrimination from other patients in the ward too manifested itself and not for the first time. On a previous day the woman in the adjacent bed had summoned a nurse, who after a whispered conversation had helped her move to as far away as possible and partly drawn the cubicle curtains. When the woman's husband visited in the afternoon there was more whispering before the curtain went even further, after both of them had given us looks compliant with their getting something on a shoe.

A later resident of that bed likewise chose to position her wheelchair firmly with its back to us each day, so that sat in it, she could presumably make believe this dreadful spectacle didn't exist. Even during the first week I had sought to assist the worried husband of another patient, after hearing a doctor loudly mention the benefit of a nasal spray he would now prescribe. It was one I knew to be very good, through lengthy use under prescription. Later on I quietly told him that when convenient I would like a word, for what I had to say would help him.

From that moment on he ignored me, supposing perhaps that I was about to proffer him a religious pamphlet, or endeavour to talk him into some dodgy investment. He would have felt better, knowing that what the doctor was prescribing would bring his wife relief. What is it with these people? Dementia even today is unfortunately still a very dirty word, despite all the publicity. One might as well have leprosy, or the plague. No matter that 600,000 have it already and the number is predicted to shortly double, whether it's so-called friends, neighbours, whatever; unless they have had a family member themselves so afflicted, they - Do Not Want To Know! - Shutting what they term as these mad people completely out of their lives.

Fasten Seat Belts!

On the day of the transfer to the new abode arrival was expected to be shortly after lunch, however, true to form, it was around five thirty when the ambulance arrived at the location which had all the ingredients for a happy home in which Mary could continue until the end of her days. It was my hope that with surroundings similar to where she had spent the last two and a half years, it would have the advantage of having nurse attendance. However the first consideration was the chest infection, if only it could be conquered. Downstairs and immediately adjacent to the nursing station, her room was bright, airy, with adequate modern furnishings and praiseworthy care.

Unfortunately by that time the odds were very heavily stacked against anything but a very slow recovery, however, now under a country doctor's practice, it was immediately evident that Mary was at last being very well looked after. Medication was stripped of all except the most important items and as the hospital antibiotics ended, my request that a further course was implemented straight way, was agreed to. Likewise other treatment to ease her breathing and make her life more bearable were added.

I visited for around three consecutive days during which time Mary looked, but a shadow of the month previous. Her voice at best was either garbled, or only a whisper, but on about the second day she did convey two never to be forgotten snippets of conversation. One comprised just four words "I like it here". That warmed my heart so, so, much, seeing I had gone through such agony to get her somewhere really nice. Somewhere which she deserved, for she had been without exception the most perfect love and wife that any man would wish for. Mary was where even she now realised was somewhere admirably befitting.

It was clean, decent, homelike with sunshine at the window, in an obviously caring environment and she knew it! The other three words you might quickly guess, but this time they would be the last words that I would hear Mary say and these were - I love YOU!; with heavy accent on that last word. On other and subsequent days, Mary's lips and teeth remained tightly closed whenever food, drink, or medication was offered. Even I, no matter what I tried, or said could not persuade Mary to awake from some kind of deep sleep and partake of them.

I played her favourite music and sat beside the bed, while those wide open yet seemingly 'unseeing' eyes although they were focused directly on my face; often gave no recognition as to her understanding of who I was, but never the less wanted that presence. I did not, could not stop telling her how much I loved her, for I understand that hearing is the last function of the body to cease functioning. There was, however, a few brief instances where half a smile featured to confirm this.

Those hours were precious, but a further cruel twist of fate would determine I would be robbed of around a week through snowfall, but principally due to my incurring about the worst water infection I had had in all thirty years of prostate related infections. Enquiring by phone as to how she was, I was told that on rare occasions Mary would talk and include myself in the conversation, also on occasion would eat small amounts of food, but the crackle in her throat continued though diminished slightly. There were I learnt several epileptic fits of varying magnitude. Told one evening that a doctor had been called as a result, I waited long minutes to know the outcome, for no way did I want her to return to hospital. As much as this had been agreed with the nursing home and various forms had been completed in regard to 'end of life' requirements and wishes.

In no way was it anything resembling a Liverpool Pathway. That concept I cannot abide, for Mary weaker as she was by the day, was being given the best chance possible to overthrow the infection, if only that were possible. Her three nurses, one English, a South African and a Greek, I knew to be thoughtful, caring and efficient. This gave me great cause to be optimistic and there of course was the comfort of prayer. Not much I'm afraid on my part, for beset with the trials of keeping going in increasing years and circumstances of recent days that had been overwhelming; I now relied on others.

Whilst with Mary in hospital on Christmas Day a gentleman appeared at my side offering a calendar. As I chose one, a phrase beneath the picture caused me to exclaim, 'Hang on, what's the catch?' It revealed him as a Baptist who takes time to visit hospitals and care homes, not to spread the word as it were, but to offer quiet conversation and comfort. Aware of the infection, then in its early stages, he said he would pray for Mary and this was no cheap gesture, for the few words he had with her revealed that they shared the loss of a child; in his case it being a devastating cot death years back.

Around fifty years ago I endured spinal problems which almost lost me my employment at a time when there was a young son and a new mortgage. Several months passed as I was stretched in hospital, with pronouncement that if there was no improvement a nasty operation would ensue, to place a piece of heel bone in my spine. Fortunately it didn't end with that and, embarrassingly, I found out that a group of people in what I will unflatteringly term a 'tin tabernacle' were praying for me. To this day I don't know who they were, or how they knew about me, but it was comforting as I survived to tell the tale.

Thus I accepted this man's offer, for he was from the country and had reared animals and worked the land. In short he had communed with nature, something which in my view allows one to have a better perspective of life. There was no miracle, not even the hoped for resurrection to former ability, but Mary did find peace in her final days and one other last facet of this story has the aspect of maybe divine intervention.

From what I have learnt, that week that I couldn't visit Mary produced more than one epileptic attack. A relatively brief one I gather scared the pants off one young gent who was attempting to feed her, while another more serious, was cause for further alarm for myself. When the phone rang one evening, I was to find that an out of hours doctor had been called, something which prompted fear of another hospital admission, despite agreement with her new country surgery that if at all possible, this should not be contemplated. I awaited the outcome as they say with bated breath.

Some twenty minutes later it was all over. Mary was fine. Two paramedics had arrived and she had just surprised one of them, by reaching up to place a kiss on his cheek in thanks for his kindness. It wasn't the first such instance either, for while Mary remained in hospital, similar blessing had been placed upon a male nurse, after she had finally received one of those all to infrequent freshen ups. As January reached its end so did Mary.

On the Thursday my antibiotics treatment was near complete and I was able to spend three to four hours by Mary's side, to play the music of one of her favourite DVDs and hold her hand and confirm again and again my love for her. She lay open mouthed, breathed with effort, but again said not a word throughout and her frame and features were one of a near to death aspect. Holding Mary's hand, was as that of a child, for the size 18 then 20 and later 22, caused by the sedentary life and copious good food, had simply evaporated away in the previous six to eight weeks.

Good-bye My Love

At somewhere after two thirty I left Mary with a kiss on the forehead. What sort of sleep it was and where she might have been, dreaming, or floating as a soul above the lifeless body I do not know. Wherever it was she was at peace. As I intimated earlier, since the admission to hospital the Alzheimer's had gone into remission. Not once had there been any urgent requests to fetch the police, to go because her husband was coming, for up to and well beyond New Year, all conversation was completely normal.

Not once was I told that I should go because her mother didn't know, or that she must leave to get the bus, because her mother was waiting. Now for all I knew Mary was already with her mother, father and the step-father she loved, but most of all perhaps reunited with her baby that she had held for so few minutes before it had to be taken away. There is no way of telling, for death remains life's greatest secret. What I do know is that little more than four hours later there was another phone call.

It was the nurse, she was concerned and had once more called the out of hours doctor. I waited unable to comprehend the outcome. At last I knew; for it was now the Greek Nurse with the news that Mary had passed away and the doctor would like to speak to me. This gentleman had spoken to me once before around a week previous when we had discussed Mary's care and medication. As the local doctor, he had apparently been returning from a function as I understand, and had decided just to drop in and see how Mary was!

At his arrival both he and the nurses were shocked, they thinking that he was answering their call and he to find his courtesy call was now one involving a death certificate. I have since found that he is a long term member of that particular country practice and, like the nursing home, portrays all that one could wish related to traditional values in this greatly changed world. This gentleman rang me again next morning regarding the exactitudes of cremation procedures and whilst conversing said that when he saw Mary two days previously, he had thought there were good grounds to see her survive the infection and live to enjoy her new abode in comfort for some time.

It was not to be, however, even though the body had as it were closed down significantly, she had remained so a full week until my return and only after seeing me for one last time, given up and slipped away. It could of course have been any minute of the previous week that the end came, but it was not. Maybe, just maybe those prayers for us both enabled it, but coupled to the fact that when speech was all but gone Mary did say those two short, but very important sentences; it really does make you wonder. I wonder too how things might have different, if only fate, or whatever had made me choose to enquire down that country lane first of all? It would have reduced Mary's time in that hospital by at least three weeks and maybe, maybe, she could have lasted longer and we enjoyed a few more precious hours together.

It would have been even better and this a most important aspect of this tale, if the care home manager had been willing to take Mary back on the understanding that nursing home care should be sourced by myself; those two months of hell for us both would not have occurred. My grief at her passing is all the more poignant in the light of those happenings and even yesterday I was to learn that her 'flat' had remained empty. So, tragically at the beginning of December, that doctor had set in motion a train of events which were destined to end Mary's life!

Did Mary know she wasn't long for this world and was the reluctance to eat and drink an obvious sign that she had had enough, upon reaching her 87th birthday just ahead of Christmas? One can only guess. Some months after Mary and I wed, my father died in a residential home and a couple of days before that event, he had told my first wife it wouldn't be long. He wasn't a religious man by any means, but he said that early one evening, 'He' had stood by the door and told him he wasn't quite ready, but his time was coming!

Mary too, on about the last day in hospital, had deteriorated to the extent that she said almost nothing while I was with her for some seven hours. It had been a demoralising day for me and I could not, but think of the fact, that going into hospital so unnecessarily had destroyed everything. She lay in bed looking more dead than alive, until somewhere around six o'clock ahead of supper arriving, something very strange, even dramatic happened.

With her face turned upward and towards the wall that flanked her bed space, she started to cry out loud enough for everyone to hear. Her arm was urgently raised, desperately reaching out to grasp something, or someone she could see, but the words that came from her lips with such energy truly amazed me. For no less than five, or six times it was 'baby', 'baby', followed by around ten calls of 'Betty', 'Betty', 'Betty', then silence returned. I certainly knew the relevance of 'baby', for many years before I became the mainstay of her life and as I have said, Mary had only been able to hold her only child in her arms for brief minutes, before it was taken away!

What followed though was the greatest surprise, for Betty was the name of the lady next door who had died of cancer around October 2010. The relationship wasn't close, only cross garden conversation and a rare visit for tea. The affinity they shared though was not only of near neighbours, but that both had developed their original and respective misfortune at the same time. That person had not been mentioned by either of us for much more than two years, for with Mary's memory loss, she wouldn't have remembered her any more than our house, garden, or anything else of our time together.

It was more than strange and there was no earthly reason for that sudden outburst, which because of its volume and urgency, stopped all conversation in the ward. We shall never know, but as with my father's experience, it was perhaps a vision beyond her dementia and even this world. I know that only days previously she had met that lady who she had not seen since our wedding day, eighteen years previous. Seeing her face had reminded her of her name, despite all those years elapsing and the onset of dementia.

Those urgent calls of "baby" and "Betty" from Mary could only have been provoked by seeing the two faces and for no other reason. I remain convinced of this, even though of course I saw nothing. Many times since, I have asked myself why I didn't ask her about it, either immediately after the event, or in the days that followed. All I can say is that I felt overwhelmed, in being privileged to witness something intensely private. Not of this world, but of the next ...

I now complete and proof read this tale as I wait for the funeral. Making the arrangements and completing the required notifications has taken up my time and to a degree stopped me concentrating too much, on how different my life will be from now on. Almost without exception the notes and sympathy cards have included the words 'Lovely Lady', because that is exactly what Mary was. To meet her, marry her and enjoy those happy years together was indeed a supreme privilege. In the weeks that follow the funeral, I will meet with the vicar at the family grave where her mother and father's remains are.

To the accompaniment of prayers, a sod will be removed and her ashes placed where she wished them to be. Later, at some as yet unknown time, my son will likewise place my ashes there also. It is what Mary wanted and what I heartily agreed to. As such it will complete the earthly aspect of our union. Further than that, who knows? What I do know, is that if we had ever talked about death, I had always said my own idea of heaven, would be that we could live together forever, but in regard to that, we will just have to wait and see!

In due course, I was to take upon myself the making of the casket for Mary's ashes and when the day arrived, it was myself who placed it in the family grave with her mother and father as she had wished. There, however, remains a legacy to Mary's final demise, in that whatever that infection was and the initial signs to the contrary; it has evidently taken root within myself. No doubt this is due to my increasing age, combined with a residual weakness stemming from a childhood of Bronchitis and Asthma. Thus any hope of assuming anything like a normal routine, is now hampered by a continuing lung condition, which to date and having had all the routine tests, is as yet without either exact diagnosis, or any cure.

The last words in this tale are, however, Mary's - My having arranged that her savings will now ensure that children can enjoy travel from the steam age for many years to come, her possessions likewise went to a good cause. Clearing almost everything and including some from myself, around 24 bags and boxes went off to a charity that concentrates upon help for Carers. A few days subsequent to this, I picked up a note pad by the phone in the bedroom. It seemed unused, but on one page it had just five words, which obviously originated from the days following Mary's initial diagnosis.

Obviously in some distress, even desperation; she must have rung her doctor ever hopeful that there might be some salvation! One can only imagine her feelings at that time, for even with cancer there remains some hope, but obviously then in total shock, Mary had simply written:

"The Doctor can do nothing!"

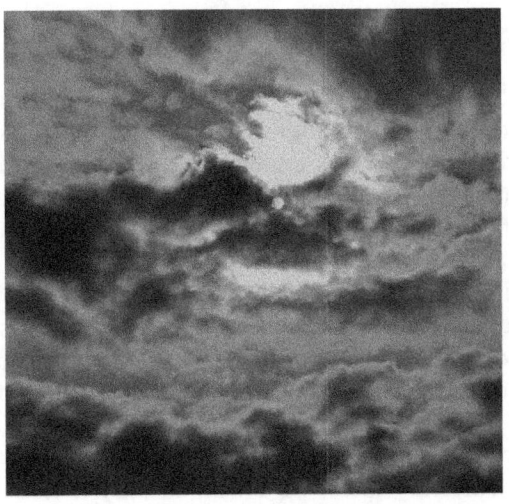

Finale

What then needs to be done? ...

... to ease the burden for Carers.

What might have made things different?

Realisation on the part of the Authorities that Dementia demands a higher entitlement of assistance to the Carer, especially as dependant on the disease's nature, it might produce the situations I have described, which leave one traumatised.

I think the most important thing is for the Authorities to recognise that where there are only a husband and wife involved, the greatest need is for the Carer to have a minimum of two three hour periods of respite each week. This need is greater of course for those aged in their 70s and 80s who tire far more easily and who therefore are less patient in difficulties.

I currently know of a woman only a stone's throw away whose husband resides either in bed, or, in a wheelchair. All she has been offered in the way of care is someone coming in to wash and dress him. That service is fine for those living alone, or for instance for a short period after leaving hospital; however the woman I speak of doesn't need that type of help, because people coming in at various times during the day only disrupts her obviously busy routine. Surely the finance which is available for a week of washing and dressing, can be used instead for a minimum three hours of respite.

Once Dementia is diagnosed, I believe the local GP should maintain regular contact with the Carer. This can easily be monthly by phone at least, to ascertain the stress levels present. Likewise the Surgery in question should arrange some method of flagging up the Carer on patient's records. Should this be done, issues of medication, appointments and other relevant matters, will be dealt with more speedily and thus considerably ease the Carer's role.

Again in regard to doctors, I'm sorry; but in my experience there isn't enough knowledge of Dementia as yet in this profession. I know that one bad apple as is well-known, can cloud your view; but those cases I quoted where the attitude equated to 'hard luck, you better get on with it', was so, so out of tune with the help and understanding of the psychiatrist; that one could only shudder at the ignorance displayed.

Social Services, which to myself equated to being very unsociable and of very little service. Well, they require a great deal more training where Dementia is concerned. Also, if someone quickly says they are well-trained, then there's something wrong with the training! First and foremost the arrogant attitude needs to go, for dishing out orders and faulting one's efforts is totally counter-productive. Coming between Husband and Wife alienates! As for these 'Best Decisions' these more than anything, are the ultimate in patronising behaviour. To me it's a bit like 'You're a naughty boy, I'm going to smack your bottom'! Bright young things too, with no experience of life are a disaster. I know everyone needs the chance to learn, but not with Dementia they don't, a longish probationary period with a senior member of staff is very much needed.

Where the Care Homes are concerned, there are several points to make. One is living the decline of one's loved one every day and in my case, I asked three times at least if it was considered that Nursing Care was about to be relevant? Rather than be told that things should stay as they were and then get dropped in it as I was, change is required. If notice had been served and I was given time to make those enquiries, a smooth transition could have taken place, minus the subsequent loss of life.

My own judgement was that the onset of epilepsy was when the one to one care was insufficient, so why didn't trained staff realise it? As for the Care Home I visited with that much proclaimed expertise in Dementia, yet didn't want its other guests disturbed! For heaven's sake, Dementia and Alzheimer's in particular, is a behavioural condition. It's no good just producing a seven star luxury home, for real quality Care and understanding, was found up that narrow country lane!

In general: Someone who has been in a Care Home, especially for a number of years, has been in a closed environment away from the normal every day infections. As such a Doctor should realise that unless the need to enter hospital is urgent, more harm may be done than good by his, or her action.

Hospitals and Care Homes apparently have a reputation for harbouring germs, in other words you should never take a baby to either, I was told! Thus when they receive a Dementia patient, they of all people should know that by putting them in a normal ward, they are placing them in immediate risk. The very nature of their debility means too, that they will require far more in the way of nursing and assistance, so where at all possible the aim should be that to protect them, such patients are placed in a small sub ward away from general visiting routines.

The Population too, needs to learn more about Dementia and to do that Government should take the lead. People with Dementia are not daft, far from it. They are the same as everyone else, but their ailment disturbs the brain, the mind, call it what you will and although this is a handicap, in no way are they the same as the Mentally Handicapped. In hindsight, the fault of the two Care Homes I visited which carried a well-known name, was that their repellent conditions displayed primarily, a non-understanding of the difference between Alzheimer's and one being mentally handicapped.

My Alzheimer's wife knew when she did something wrong and if told of it, would apologise for it profusely. My guess is, that this may be a simple indicator of what differentiates these two categories. Those Care Homes needed to emulate the 'country lanes' ethic of Dementia patients needing what Mary had enjoyed previously. This was namely 'Home' like surroundings, but with much more help, as its later stage was complicated by the onset of epilepsy.

The Government already mentioned above, needs to understand that this scourge is apparently increasing at an alarming rate, so where finance is concerned, additional resources should be allocated to aid communities country wide. At the moment it's concentrating on planning a cap on Care charges. One's assets are now quoted and they take house that you have worked for and hope to pass on to your children will be forcefully sacrificed. Why? Does this same rule apply if instead of owning a house, you pay rent, but have a large mobile home, yacht and some very expensive objects d'art, do they take them as well? We are fighting a war against Dementia and Cancer within society. The casualty rate is increasing! Your home is not taken away in a war with another nation, so why now? All that is the totally wrong approach, what is really needed is that Care in the Community really is that and no individual has to undergo what I had, with only minimal help and a great deal of aggravation throughout.

Finally the various support organisations. A difficult one this, for in no way do I want to stop people donating. My current opinion is conditioned solely by my own experience. This being so I will talk of charities and while in no way downgrading other maladies, Dementia and Cancer are the two greatest challenges in today's world. Dementia however is likely to engender the greatest effect long term, as it now strikes even younger persons, as well as those who have reached their later years and are less robust.

This being so and with the reported cases swelling by the day, those two conditions cry out for Government action. Far too much aid is currently directed at powerful countries on the other side of the world and highly suspect regimes in Africa in particular. If Care in the Community is to really work and thereby ease a burden on society which ever increases, an improved and highly efficient system will need greater Government funding. Why? Because it has become a truly National problem.

Co-related to this, charities in general are required to be far more transparent, for past investigation has produced alarming figures to apparently show that only a small percentage of money contributed, often actually ends up where the givers hope it will. As perhaps leader in the public's eyes, the Alzheimer's Society empathises that money is needed for research and it most certainly is, but surely research by a combination of Universities and the big drug companies (who let's face it have the most to gain), is already substantial. The old concept of 'throw enough mud at a wall and some of it will stick', is wasteful. Why not a Royal Commission to promptly determine the exact situation, this being also very much a guide to at what level new and major Government funding should be!

Once this was completed, the Alzheimer's Society and other leading organisations, would be able to concentrate exclusively on using their donations, to help those directly affected and in particular the husband and wife Carers who are of advanced years. It is a fact that with more help I could have managed much longer. Even a period of true respite can recharge the batteries as it were and you return to the fray renewed. Also contrary to the expressed view, a change of location, e.g into care temporarily, or even briefly to hospital, can result in an amelioration of the condition, which even if of short duration becomes a real Godsend for both the patient and their Carer.

I rest my Case.

A Postscript

(1) The Hospital - refuses point blank to ask visitors to leave, however obvious their signs of infection are. Likewise it has said that patients coming from a sheltered environment, can only be placed in a normal ward.

> ... Callous and frustrating!

(2) The 'Posh' care home - that 'could not have its other guests disturbed', despite supposedly knowing everything there was to know about Dementia; has just been awarded not one, but two awards.

> ... Sickening!

(3) Another 'Posh' care home only opened a matter of weeks back, has already received an award.

> ... Unbelievable!

(4) The Private Company - which took over the County Council care homes on 1 December 2012 - has staff shortages and worse. It introduced new contracts, redundancy packages and lower rates of pay for all new employees.

> ... Typical and certainly not the way to get the best quality staff

(5) The County Council Carers Service - (after 2½ years), still sends me its literature. Full of events for Carers to attend, but not a word about how cover would be found to take over.

> ... Pathetic!

(6) The Local Authority - (also after 2½ years) and their official's visit report which I retain, still had me recorded as a Carer, Council Tax wise.
... Ludicrous!

(7) The Care Home Manager, I learn, has not only consistently lied to her staff and Social Services, that I took Mary away from the care home. The Hospital's ward matron and doctors involved, however, know differently! As a further demonstration of her true nature, the 'Thank You' letter destined for her staff was destroyed, rather than its well-deserved content of appreciation be displayed!
... Any comment here, is unprintable.

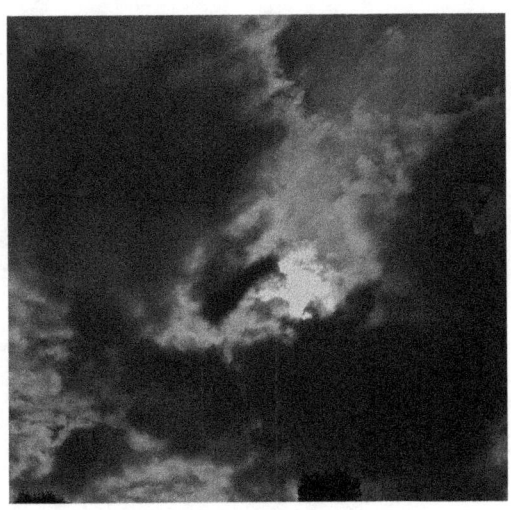

www.ingramcontent.com/pod-product-compliance
Lightning Source LLC
Chambersburg PA
CBHW071422170526
45165CB00001B/364